# Update of Today's Facial Skin Rejuvenation Technology

*Editor*

RICHARD D. GENTILE

# FACIAL PLASTIC SURGERY CLINICS OF NORTH AMERICA

www.facialplastic.theclinics.com

*Consulting Editor*
J. REGAN THOMAS

February 2020 • Volume 28 • Number 1

**ELSEVIER**

1600 John F. Kennedy Boulevard • Suite 1800 • Philadelphia, Pennsylvania, 19103-2899

http://www.theclinics.com

**FACIAL PLASTIC SURGERY CLINICS OF NORTH AMERICA Volume 28, Number 1**
**February 2020 ISSN 1064-7406, ISBN-13: 978-0-323-69596-1**

Editor: Jessica McCool
Developmental Editor: Laura Kavanaugh

*Facial Plastic Surgery Clinics of North America* (ISSN 1064-7406) is published quarterly by Elsevier Inc., 360 Park Avenue South, New York, NY 10010-1710. Months of issue are February, May, August, and November. Business and Editorial Offices: 1600 John F. Kennedy Blvd., Suite 1800, Philadelphia, PA 19103-2899. Periodicals postage paid at New York, NY, and additional mailing offices. Subscription prices are $408.00 per year (US individuals), $692.00 per year (US institutions), $454.00 per year (Canadian individuals), $861.00 per year (Canadian institutions), $535.00 per year (foreign individuals), $861.00 per year (foreign institutions), $100.00 per year (US students), $100.00 per year (Canadian students), and $255.00 per year (foreign students). Foreign air speed delivery is included in all *Clinics* subscription prices. All prices are subject to change without notice. POSTMASTER: Send address changes to *Facial Plastic Surgery Clinics*, Elsevier Health Sciences Division, Subscription Customer Service, 3251 Riverport Lane, Maryland Heights, MO 63043. **Customer service: 1-800-654-2452 (US and Canada); 1-314-447-8871 (outside US and Canada); Fax: 314-447-8029; E-mail: journalscustomerservice-usa@elsevier.com (for print support); journalsonlinesupport-usa@elsevier.com (for online support).**

*Reprints*. For copies of 100 or more of articles in this publication, please contact the Commercial Reprints Department, Elsevier Inc., 360 Park Avenue South, New York, NY 10010-1710. Tel.: 212-633-3874; Fax: 212-633-3820; E-mail: reprints@elsevier.com.

*Facial Plastic Surgery Clinics of North America* is covered in *MEDLINE/PubMed* (*Index Medicus*).

# Contributors

## CONSULTING EDITOR

**J. REGAN THOMAS, MD**
Professor, Facial Plastic and Reconstructive
Surgery, Department of Otolaryngology–Head
and Neck Surgery, Northwestern University
Feinberg School of Medicine, Chicago, Illinois,
USA

## EDITOR

**RICHARD D. GENTILE, MD, MBA**
Medical Director Facial Plastic Surgery, Gentile
Facial Plastic Surgery and Aesthetic Laser
Center, Youngstown, Ohio, USA; Staff
Physician, Facial Plastic Surgery, Cleveland
Clinic Akron General Hospital, Akron, Ohio,
USA

## AUTHORS

**DANA ALESSA, MD**
Assistant Professor, King Saud bin Abdulaziz
University for Health Sciences (KSAU-HS),
Riyadh, Saudi Arabia

**MACRENE ALEXIADES, MD, PhD**
Associate Clinical Professor, Yale School of
Medicine, New Haven, Connecticut, USA;
Adjunct Clinical Professor, University of Athens
Sygros Hospital, Athens, Greece; Founder and
Director, Dermatology and Laser Surgery
Center of New York, New York, USA

**KAETE A. ARCHER, MD**
Assistant Professor, Columbia University,
Aesthetic Institute of Manhattan for Facial and
Plastic Surgery, New York, New York, USA

**ERNEST A. AZZOPARDI, MD, MSc Surg.
PhD, MRCSEd, MRCSEng (Ad Eudem), Dip
spec laser, FRSB, FRCSEd (Plast)**
Consultant Plastic Surgeon and Laser
Specialist, Laserplast SrL StP, Milano, Italy;
R&D Department, Swansea Bay University
Health Board, Welsh Centre for Burns and
Plastic Surgery, Morriston Hospital, Swansea,
Wales, United Kingdom

**PATRICK BITTER Jr, MD, FAAD**
Founder and CEO, Dermatology, Advanced
Aesthetic Dermatology, Los Gatos, California,
USA

**JASON D. BLOOM, MD, FACS**
Adjunct Assistant Professor, Department of
Otorhinolaryngology-Head and Neck Surgery,
University of Pennsylvania, Philadelphia,
Pennsylvania, USA; Bloom Facial Plastic
Surgery, Bryn Mawr, Pennsylvania,
USA

**PAUL J. CARNIOL, MD**
Clinical Professor, Department of
Otolaryngology, Rutgers New Jersey Medical
School, Summit, New Jersey, USA

**MATTEO TRETTI CLEMENTONI, MD**
Consultant Plastic Surgeon and Laser
Specialist, Laserplast SrL StP, Milano,
Italy

**DEBRA FROST, MPH**
Los Angeles, California, USA

**RICHARD D. GENTILE, MD, MBA**
Medical Director, Facial Plastic Surgery,
Gentile Facial Plastic Surgery and Aesthetic
Laser Center, Youngstown, Ohio, USA; Staff
Physician, Facial Plastic Surgery, Cleveland
Clinic Akron General Hospital, Akron, Ohio,
USA

**J. DAVID HOLCOMB, MD**
Holcomb – Kreithen Plastic Surgery and
MedSpa, Sarasota, Florida, USA

**KIAN KARIMI, MD, FACS**
Rejuva Medical Aesthetics, Los Angeles,
California, USA

**DEVINDER S. MANGAT, MD, FACS**
Facial Plastic and Reconstructive Surgeon,
Mangat Plastic Surgery, Edwards, Colorado,
USA

**BENJAMIN CARL MARCUS, MD**
Director of Facial Plastic Surgery, Department
of Otolaryngology, University of Wisconsin-
Madison, Madison, Wisconsin, USA

**J.D. McCOY, NMD**
Medical Director, Aesthetic Medicine, Contour
Medical, Gilbert, Arizona, USA

**LAURA ROMANA MOTTA, MD**
Consultant Dermatologist, Laserplast SrL StP,
Milano, Italy

**LAWRENCE S. MOY, MD**
Los Angeles, California, USA

**STEPHANIE MOY, BS**
Los Angeles, California, USA

**VALERIO PEDRELLI, MD**
Consultant Dermatologist, Laserplast SrL StP,
Milano, Italy

**PAOLO PONTINI, MD**
Consultant Dermatologist, Laserplast SrL StP,
Milano, Italy

**AUNNA POURANG, MD**
Department of Dermatology, University of
California, Irvine, Irvine, California, USA

**HELENA ROCKWELL, BSc**
University of California, San Diego, School of
Medicine, La Jolla, California, USA

**RAMINDER SALUJA, MD, FAAO, FASLMS**
Saluja Cosmetic and Laser Center, Private
Practice, Huntersville, North Carolina, USA

**SIDNEY J. STARKMAN, MD**
Facial Plastic and Reconstructive Surgeon,
Starkman Facial Plastic Surgery, Scottsdale,
Arizona, USA

**WILLIAM H. TRUSWELL, MD, FACS**
Clinical Instructor, Division of Otolaryngology–
Head and Neck Surgery, University of
Connecticut School of Medicine, Farmington,
Connecticut, USA; President, American Board
of Facial Plastic and Reconstructive Surgery,
Past President, American Academy of Facial
Plastic and Reconstructive Surgery, Senior
Advisor European Board of Facial Plastic and
Reconstructive Surgery, Senior Advisor
International Board for Certification in Facial
Plastic and Reconstructive Surgery, Private
Practice, Easthampton, Massachusetts, USA

**GIOVANNA ZACCARIA, MD**
Consultant Dermatologist, Laserplast SrL StP,
Milano, Italy

# Contents

The use of microneedling with or without radiofrequency continues to expand in aesthetics. There are now many different devices available that have multiple indications, unique protocols, and low side effect profiles.

Microneedle radiofrequency (RF) is a breakthrough in targeting skin laxity and rhytids that provides direct in situ delivery, impedance measurements, temperature measurements, energy delivery controls, and targeting of various skin depths to achieve desired clinical outcomes. Microneedle RF controls penetration depth and delivery to specified temperatures and impedance measurements, ensuring significantly improved efficacy in the treatment of mild-to-moderate rhytids and skin laxity of the face and neck, and cellulite and laxity on other body sites. Combining microneedle RF with dermal fillers and neuromodulators may be used to further improve clinical outcomes and achieve high patient satisfaction.

Fractional $CO_2$ procedures are an established, safe and effective armamentarium for managing skin rejuvenation and scarring. Very short-pulse-duration devices offer a very high ablated volume/ablated surface ratio, inducing a controlled thermal damage. With this kind of device, each procedure can be customized on the features of the skin of each patient. The same device can be used to treat severe burn scars. With a very deep fractional procedure on a scar tissue, immediate relaxation of the tension and retraction forces may be obtained, and downstream, improvements are related more to the activation of a molecular cascade. The authors review the state-of-the-art, in the use of fractioned $CO_2$ laser technology for aesthetic and scar remodelling indications.

Pulsed light has proven its usefulness, effectiveness and versatility in treating a multitude of skin problems, delaying skin aging, maintaining healthy skin, and as an adjunct to a cosmetic surgical practive for non-invasive skin rejuvenation and treating postsurgical scars. Practitioners contemplating adding a pulsed light device to their practice should choose a device that has at least four important features: a large spot size, variable-sized smaller spot adaptors, pulse rates of at least 1 pulse per second and a range of cutoff filters from 515 nm to 695 nm to treat most skin types. Training to master the use of a pulsed light device is essential to obtain consistent and predictable results with minimal complications.

In the 2000s, there was a significant expansion in technology that was described as "nonablative." These devices featured several different wavelengths and technologies. What they shared in common was the goal of delivering improvement in skin appearance while minimizing downtime and complications. Most of the "less-invasive" devices relied on the advent of fractional technology. This was the design feat of having multiple very small laser pulses delivered in a gridlike fashion and allowed for a mosaic of treated and untreated skin. With islands of healthy skin next to treated skin, the healing process was thought to be more rapid.

With modern medicine increasing both the average life span and quality of life, there has been a greater demand for treatment of age-related skin changes. As many new options in skin resurfacing are developed annually, it is chemical peeling that has withstood the trials of time and scrutiny. The different variations of chemoexfoliation have been used for rhytids, actinic damage, lentigos, and dyschromias. This article describes the most recent knowledge about chemical peeling, and exposes previously accepted yet incorrect dogmas. Chemical peeling, when practiced with knowledge and good technique, can yield excellent results in skin rejuvenation.

Beauty of the face is dependent on many factors, measurable and intangible. The concept of a beautiful face varies from era to era and culture to culture. Maintenance, improvement, and creation of beautiful skin benefit from procedures, prescriptive topicals, cosmeceuticals, and cosmetics. Current science and art are children of the efforts of previous practitioners of past generations. A thorough understanding of how the skin ages is necessary for choosing the appropriate therapeutic approach to halt and reverse signs of aging. The concept of beauty, history of skin treatments, skin anatomy, aging process of skin, and prescriptive skin care products are examined herein.

 Video content accompanies this article at http://www.facialplastic.theclinics.com.

Nitrogen plasma skin regeneration (PSR) initiated the use of cold atmospheric plasma (CAP) in skin rejuvenation over a decade ago. Helium gas CAP is already in widespread use worldwide for many surgical applications, whereas its use in skin rejuvenation is now emerging as a viable tool for treatment of facial rhytidosis. Animal studies comparing these CAPs suggest that observed differences in skin tissue interaction result from differences in plasma generation and in energy deposition wherein greater skin tissue contraction observed with helium PSR may result from its unique bimodal energy deposition and more complete full field treatment of the tissue.

Energy-based skin rejuvenation has, like other forms of aesthetic treatments, the capability of achieving desirable end results. These end results must be balanced with the degree and duration of morbidity, which affect recovery from treatment. Renuvion skin resurfacing protocols include a free hand approach and we describe our preferred approach of pulsing and fractionating the helium plasma resurfacing energy.

Picosecond laser technology was cleared by Food and Drug Administration in 2012 and enhanced our ability to clear both benign pigmentation and dermal ink through a photomechanical impact created in the tissue. This impact created is greater than comparative nanotechnology and can be accomplished with lower fluences and smaller pulse durations. The addition of a diffractive lens array (FOCUS lens) has created a new category in skin rejuvenation by stimulating elastin and collagen through photomechanical and photoacoustic effects and not only through traditional photothermal tissue effects.

 Video content accompanies this article at http://www.facialplastic.theclinics.com.

One of the greatest challenges in the progression of aesthetic medicine lies in providing treatments with long-term results that are also minimally invasive and safe. Keeping up with this demand are developments in autologous therapies such as adipose-derived stem cells, stromal vascular fraction, microfat, nanofat, and platelet therapies, which are being shown to deliver satisfactory results. Innovations in more traditional cosmetic therapies, such as botulinum toxin, fillers, and thread lifts, are even more at the forefront of the advancement in aesthetics. Combining autologous therapies with traditional noninvasive methods can ultimately provide patients with more effective rejuvenation options.

Facial aging is a combination of descent of facial tissues, atrophy of fat compartments, bony remodeling, and photoaging/chronologic changes of the skin. Cutaneous photoaging is due to UV-A and UV-generated free radicals that cause DNA mutations, structural and enzymatic protein alterations, and lipid peroxidation. Many of the histologic and histochemical changes associated with photoaging can be reversed with laser resurfacing. Post laser resurfacing wound care is important for optimizing recovery. There is some controversy over the use of prophylactic antibiotics.

The process of obtaining blood biologics, including platelet-rich plasma (PRP) and platelet-rich fibrin (PRF), can be complicated and expensive and is influenced by many vendors and proprietary techniques. The indications for PRP/PRF use remain controversial, and complicated or expensive modes of generating this biologic may lead to many facial plastic surgeons to pass on the use of these potentially useful agents. The lack of standardization of PRP procurement also has led to difficulties in assessing clinical efficacy and comparing study protocols.

Photodynamic therapy is the combination of the initial application of a photosensitive chemical on the skin and then using typically a blue filter light of varying spectrums. This treatment protocol has been more useful and functional than other chemical peels and lasers for a variety of conditions. There has been efficacy in antiviral treatments, such as herpetic lesions; malignant cancers of the head and neck; and lung, bladder, and skin cancers. It has been tested for prostate cancers, cervical cancer, colorectal cancer, lung cancer, breast cancer, esophageal cancer, stomach cancer, pancreatic cancer, vaginal cancer, gliomas, and erythroplasia of Queyrat.

# FACIAL PLASTIC SURGERY CLINICS
# OF NORTH AMERICA

---

### SERIES OF RELATED INTEREST

*Clinics in Plastic Surgery*
https://www.plasticsurgery.theclinics.com/
*Otolaryngologic Clinics*
https://www.oto.theclinics.com/

---

**THE CLINICS ARE AVAILABLE ONLINE!**
Access your subscription at:
www.theclinics.com

# Foreword
# Update on Facial Skin Rejuvenation Technology

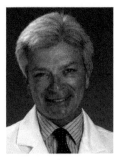

J. Regan Thomas, MD
*Consulting Editor*

Recent years have provided multiple modalities being promoted for improvement of facial appearance, including facial rhytid removal or smoothing, facial lesion correction, scar improvement, and general tightening and skin rejuvenation. Evaluation of the effectiveness of these techniques in addition to insightful selection of the appropriate equipment and treatment technology can be challenging to the contemporary facial plastic surgeon. This issue of *Facial Plastic Surgery Clinics of North America* is organized to address these questions and help educate the reader regarding the types of treatment results that can be expected from a variety of technologies and techniques.

Dr Gentile as guest editor has organized a thorough and extensive overview of the multiple facial skin treatments and the technology to provide those treatments for this issue. The article authors represent experienced and insightful expertise for multiple treatments and technical applications for this important component of facial plastic surgery practice. The articles cover expertise ranging from laser modalities and other energy-based treatments to chemical peel approaches and microneedle skin rejuvenation. New approaches to gaining the effects of stem cell use and platelet-rich fibrin are described as well as suggestions for skin care products.

These patient care and rejuvenation approaches have been rapidly growing and frequently changing in recent years. Dr Gentile and the selected group of contributing authors for this issue provide an outstanding update of this evolving component of facial plastic surgery practice for the readership. Their insights, experience, and expertise make a valuable contribution available to the facial plastic surgery literature.

J. Regan Thomas, MD
Department of Otolaryngology–Head and Neck Surgery
Northwestern University School of Medicine
675 North Saint Clair Street
Suite 15-200
Chicago, IL 60611, USA

*E-mail address:*
Regan.Thomas@nm.org

https://doi.org/10.1016/j.fsc.2019.10.001
1064-7406/20/

facialplastic.theclinics.com

# Preface

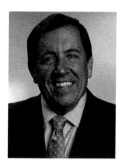

Richard D. Gentile, MD, MBA
*Editor*

Having beautiful skin has been a constant desire through the ages, and the history of skin improvement, including cosmetics, dates to ancient Egypt nearly 6000 years ago.[1] My interest in skin care started with my residency training at Baylor College of Medicine. At that time, most commercial skin-care improvement products existed in cosmetics, and not much was available for prescription skin-care and medical practice. The laser era was in its infancy. Retin A was introduced for acne treatment in 1962 but became popular as a wrinkle therapy and has remained highly prescribed along with retinol, its milder cousin. Soon thereafter, hydroxy acid products and a litany of various products based on plant and other growth factors developed. Early in my career, I was trained in various types of chemexfoliation, and in 1994, I purchased my first laser for skin rejuvenation. This was followed by over 30 more in the years to come and a commitment to invest in the best technologies and techniques for skin rejuvenation. The devices available now are used not only above the skin but also under. In 2008, we introduced subdermal skin tightening using the SmartLipo laser, and it has led to the development of many technological developments for tightening skin from below the skin. The desire for beautiful skin has remained a constant and with it the development of the entire aesthetic and cosmetics industry. Skin rejuvenation and skin care are now practiced not only by skin-care specialists but also by nonspecialists and specialists of other medical and surgical specialties. This issue examines the many different approaches to contemporary skin rejuvenation.

I am grateful to the authors, editors, and others who have contributed to the completion of this issue of the *Facial Plastic Surgery Clinics of North America*. It has certainly been my pleasure to contribute to its publication, and I hope that it is useful to those reading to improve their efforts to help our patients with skin issues whether caused by disease, trauma, or aging.

Richard D. Gentile, MD, MBA
Gentile Facial Plastic Surgery and
Aesthetic Laser Center
821 Kentwood Suite C
Youngstown, OH 44512, USA

Facial Plastic Surgery
Cleveland Clinic Akron General Hospital
Akron, OH 44307, USA

*E-mail address:*
dr-gentile@msn.com

## REFERENCE

1. Available at: https://www.laseraway.com/news/brief-history-skincare-ages/. Accessed October 1, 2019.

Facial Plast Surg Clin N Am 28 (2020) xiii
https://doi.org/10.1016/j.fsc.2019.10.002
1064-7406/20/© 2019 Published by Elsevier Inc.

# Microneedling Options for Skin Rejuvenation, Including Non–temperature-controlled Fractional Microneedle Radiofrequency Treatments

Dana Alessa, MD[a], Jason D. Bloom, MD, FACS[b,c],*

## KEYWORDS

- Microneedling • Radiofrequency • Radiofrequency microneedling • Acne scars • Skin rejuvenation

## KEY POINTS

- Conventional microneedling and radiofrequency microneedling are considered safe and effective methods for skin rejuvenation, if performed appropriately.
- Treatments are safe for all skin types because, unlike lasers, they are chromophore blind.
- Treatments are usually well tolerated with topical anesthesia and with minimal side effects.
- The proper device selection and treatment parameters are essential keys to successful therapies.
- There are expanding indications for these devices, including but not limited to hyperhidrosis, cellulite, striae.

## INTRODUCTION

The use of microneedling for aesthetic purposes has been well studied over the years. Most of the documented work using this technology has been to study acne scars; however, its efficacy in other areas, such as surgical or traumatic scars, melasma, striae, androgenetic alopecia, and skin rejuvenation, has also been studied. Radiofrequency (RF) microneedling (RFMN) is a newer technology that has shown promising results for skin rejuvenation and acne scars and is discussed in this article.

## MECHANISM OF ACTION

Percutaneous collagen induction is the basic theory behind all forms of microneedling technology. Histologic studies have shown increased new collagen and elastin after the use of microneedling tools, such as the original Dermaroller. When using such devices, small zones of injury are created in the papillary dermis, which then undergo the wound healing process and cascade, resulting in improved scars and wrinkles. The nonablative (sparing the epidermis) nature of microneedling makes it ideal for all skin types with almost no risk for hyperpigmentation.[1]

Radiofrequency microneedling functions by delivering RF energy at a selected tissue depth using a multiple needle probe array. In general, RF devices use electromagnetic energy in order to generate heat in tissues through the rapid movement of charged particles. This heat ultimately

Disclosures: None.
[a] King Saud bin Abdulaziz University for Health Sciences (KSAU-HS), PO Box 3660, Riyadh 11481, Saudi Arabia; [b] Bloom Facial Plastic Surgery, Two Town Place, Suite 110, Bryn Mawr, PA 19010, USA; [c] Department of Otorhinolaryngology—Head & Neck Surgery, University of Pennsylvania, 3400 Civic Center Blvd, South Pavillion 3rd Floor, Philadelphia, PA 19104, USA
* Corresponding author. Bloom Facial Plastic Surgery, Two Town Place, Suite 110, Bryn Mawr, PA 19010.
*E-mail address:* drjbloom@bloomfps.com

Facial Plast Surg Clin N Am 28 (2020) 1–7
https://doi.org/10.1016/j.fsc.2019.09.001
1064-7406/20/© 2019 Elsevier Inc. All rights reserved.

leads to collagen denaturation and the shrinkage or contraction of tissue when a critical temperature is reached (65°C to 75°C).[2]

Clinical and histologic studies have shown the efficacy of transepidermal nonablative RF for tissue remodeling; neocollagenesis through collagen fibril contraction and clinical improvement was noted in the periorbital area (decreased periorbital wrinkles, improved brow position), midface/lower face (nasolabial folds, marionette lines, jowls, laxity under the chin), and neck laxity.[3–6] Histologic analysis of skin tissue treated with RFMN for acne and acne scars also showed increased collagen deposition through upregulated transforming growth factor beta, and decreased inflammatory markers such as nuclear factor-κB and interleukin-8.[7]

In contrast with lasers, which are used to target selective chromophores in tissues, RF functions by nonselective tissue heating (independent of tissue chromophores), making it safer in darker skin types.[8]

### Microneedling

The reported safety and efficacy of microneedling treatments initially made it an attractive procedure for patients looking for an effective aesthetic procedure with minimal downtime.

The tools used for these procedures include rollers and electric pen devices with disposable tips. During the treatment, the device is held perpendicularly and rolled or glided over the skin until pinpoint bleeding is appreciated. Needle penetration depths are adjusted by the provider, depending on the particular area and skin thickness to be treated, with deeper needles for thick skin and shorter needle depth for thin or delicate skin, such as the periorbital area.[9]

SkinPen (Bellus Medical) is the first US Food and Drug Administration (FDA)–cleared microneedling device for facial acne scars.

## MICRONEEDLING FOR ACNE SCARS

One of the earliest microneedling studies was done with a rolling tool (Dermaroller) that has 94 microneedles at the tip, with depth varying from 0.1 mm to 1.3 mm, depending on the amount of pressure applied to the skin. Thirty-two subjects with rolling-type acne scars received 2 treatments, 8 weeks apart. Results showed that all subjects had greatly reduced scar severity.[10]

In a randomized controlled trial of 15 subjects with acne scars, 1 side of the face served as the treatment side and received 3 microneedling treatments, whereas the other side of the face served as the control. Results showed significantly improved scars on the treatment side compared with baseline, whereas no significant change was noted on the control side.[11]

Compared with nonablative fractional laser treatment of acne scarring, 2 randomized controlled trials showed no significant difference in efficacy between microneedling alone or combined with 20% trichloroacetic acid and nonablative fractional laser (1540 nm and 1340 nm).[12,13]

Split-face controlled trials comparing microneedling alone or with vitamin C with microneedling combined with platelet-rich plasma (PRP) for acne scars showed superior results in the latter combined group (microneedling + PRP). These results are produced by the combined effects of growth factors triggered by cutaneous wounds from microneedling, as well as growth factors contained in PRP.[14–16]

## MICRONEEDLING: TRANSEPIDERMAL DRUG DELIVERY

Many studies have investigated the idea and efficacy of using microneedling as a tool to enhance drug delivery into the skin.

In a randomized controlled trial of 100 male subjects with moderate to severe androgenetic alopecia, subjects randomized to the treatment group receiving microneedling combined with the topical application of minoxidil had statistically significant superior results in hair growth compared with subjects receiving minoxidil only.[17]

A controlled trial investigating the treatment of melasma was conducted among 20 subjects who had split-face treatment; 1 side had microneedling combined with a depigmenting serum and the other side had the serum alone. The results of this study showed a statistically significant reduction in the Melasma Area and Severity Index score in the combined treatment side compared with the side treated with the serum alone.[18]

## MICRONEEDLING FOR SKIN REJUVENATION (LAXITY AND WRINKLES)

Clinical and histologic assessments were done in 10 patients who underwent 6 microneedling treatments using a Dermaroller and the results showed significant improvement in wrinkles, skin texture, and overall satisfaction as well as increased collagen and tropoelastin in biopsy specimens.[19]

Statistically significant improvement in the signs of photoaging (wrinkles, laxity, and texture) was also seen in another study using a motorized microneedling device.[20]

## Radiofrequency Microneedling

### The technology

Not all RFMN devices are equal. There are 2 different types of needle used in these devices: noninsulated microneedles delivering energy throughout the needle length, and insulated microneedles delivering energy only at the needle tip in the dermis, thus protecting the epidermis from heat and thermal damage.

Most devices deliver bipolar RF energy where the current is traveling between positive and negative electrodes on the tip, limiting the current in the treated area for a controlled distribution. With monopolar RF, the current is traveling between the active electrode tip in the treated area and a grounding electrode at a distant body location, allowing deeper or improved energy penetration.[21,22] Compared with monopolar RF, bipolar RF requires less energy and provides less energy depth penetration because of the smaller and contained area of current passage.[2]

### Some radiofrequency microneedling devices on the market

- INTRAcel (Jeisys, South Korea) device offers both monopolar and bipolar options. The tip is composed of 49 insulated microneedles with 4 needle depth options: 0.5 mm, 0.8 mm, 1.5 mm, and 2.0 mm.
- Fractora (InMode, Israel) has multiple alternatives for tips with different densities, lengths, and insulation options that function through bipolar technology: deep dermal, low-density, 3000-$\mu$m, 24-pin tip; deep and subdermal low-density, 3000-$\mu$m silicon coated 24-pin tip; and mid-dermal, high-density, 600-$\mu$m, 60-pin tip. Morpheus8 is the newest RFMN device, with deeper needle depths that spare the dermis for action in the subcutaneous adipose tissue, and 24 insulated pins with depths of more than 4000 $\mu$m.
- Intensif (Endymed, Caesarea, Israel) was the first FDA-cleared RFMN device. The needle tip has 25 noninsulated gold microneedles with needle depths ranging from 0.5 mm to 5.0 mm, power 0 W to 25 W, and pulse duration 50 to 200 milliseconds.
- INFINI (Lutronic) delivers bipolar RF energy with 49 insulated microneedles in the tip. Depths range from 0.5 mm to 3.5 mm, power 2.5 W to 50 W, and pulse duration 10 to 1000 milliseconds. Genius is Lutronic's second-generation RFMN device, with proprietary technology that allows more precise needle and energy delivery through continuous impedance monitoring for optimal treatment.
- Vivace (Cartessa) offers both insulated and noninsulated 36-microneedle tips. Depths range from 0.5 mm to 3.5 mm, power 30 W to 70 W, and pulse duration 100 to 800 milliseconds. The system also delivers LED (light-emitting diode) light at the same time with 2 options: blue light for an antibacterial effect and red light for collagen stimulation.

Table 1 shows a comparison between the devices based on a compilation of physician surveys independently conducted using a fixed survey format and defined criteria by ZALEA. These results do not reflect ZALEA's testing or opinion.

The first use of an RFMN device was studied by Hantash and colleagues[23,24] using a bipolar device that featured temperature and impedance transcription, allowing the delivery of energy at a preselected temperature and depth, respectively. Histologic evaluation of biopsy specimens showed areas of collagen denaturation (RF thermal zones) followed by dermal remodeling through neocollagenesis and neoelastogenesis.

**Table 1**
**Comparison between the devices based on a compilation of physician surveys independently conducted using a fixed survey format and defined criteria by ZALEA**

|  | INTRAcel | INFINI | Fractora | Intensif |
|---|---|---|---|---|
| ZALEA Physician Editors Rating | 4 out of 5 | 4 out of 5 | 3 out of 5 | 3 out of 5 |
| Overall Rating | 7.9 out of 10 | 7.5 out of 10 | 7.2 out of 10 | 6.3 out of 10 |
| Marketing Claims | 7.7 | 8.3 | 8.5 | 7.2 |
| Peer-reviewed Literature | 6.6 | 7.7 | 7 | 6 |
| Consistency of Results | 8.6 | 8.4 | 8.8 | 7.6 |
| Comfort Level | 8.1 | 5.1 | 3.5 | 4.2 |
| Overall Satisfaction | 8.4 | 7.8 | 8 | 6.4 |

These results do not reflect ZALEA's testing or opinion.

## RADIOFREQUENCY MICRONEEDLING FOR ACNE AND ACNE SCARS

Most of literature on RFMN to treat acne scarring was in patients with dark skin types, given the increased safety profile and lower risk for postinflammatory hyperpigmentation (PIH) with such treatments.

In 2 of the studies that investigated the efficacy and safety of RFMN for acne scars in subjects with skin types III to V, the assessments were done using the Goodman and Barron's Global Qualitative Acne Scarring System (1, macular; 2, mild; 3, moderate; 4, severe). One had 31 subjects with mixed types of acne scars and these patients had 4 treatments separated 6 weeks apart, using the INFINI device. Three months after the last treatment was the final evaluation of results. In the 14 subjects with a baseline of grade 4, 12 (85.71%) showed a 2-grade improvement and 2 (14.28%) showed a 1-grade improvement. Of the remaining 17 subjects with a grade 3 baseline score, 13 (76.47%) showed a 2-grade improvement and 4 (23.52%) showed a 1-grade improvement.[25] The other study had 19 subjects who received 3 monthly treatments with the Intensif device. An evaluation of the treatments occurred 1 month following 3 separate treatment sessions. Eleven

of 19 patients (57.9%) had at least 1-grade improvement and, 3 months following the third session, 9 patients were again evaluated and all showed at least 1-grade improvement. Nine subjects (47.4%) also showed improvement in facial dyschromia.[26]

Encountered side effects of these procedures included pain, erythema, edema, and PIH, all of which were transient (**Fig. 1**).

Further acne-related research, investigating the improvement in active acne lesions and acne-related postinflammatory erythema with RFMN, was performed in darker-skinned patients. The results of those studies support the evidence that treatment with RFMN produced decreased inflammation. The results of 3 INTRAcel treatments on 25 subjects with moderate to severe acne showed a 90.11% decrease in inflammatory acne, a 76.46% decrease in noninflammatory acne, and a 36.99% decrease in sebum excretion.[27] The INFINI device was used in a related study for acne-related postinflammatory erythema in which 25 subjects in the treatment group receiving 2 RFMN treatments were compared with 27 subjects in the control group receiving oral or topical therapy. Compared with the control group, the treatment group showed statistically significant improvement in

## ACNE SCARS

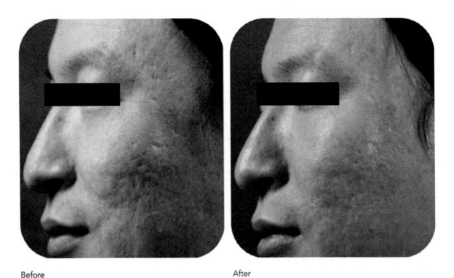

Before                     After

**Fig. 1.** Before and 1 month after 3 INTRAcel treatments for acne scars. (*Courtesy of* Jeisys Corporation, Seoul, KR; with permission.)

the investigators' global assessment score, as well in objective assessment of erythema with both photometric device and digital software. Histologic studies showed decreased vascularity, inflammation, and inflammatory markers in the treatment group.[28] Side effects reported were pain, erythema, bleeding, scaling, and crusting, which all resolved in a few days to 1 week (**Fig. 2**).

Compared with transepidermal bipolar RF, a randomized clinical trial of 20 subjects with mild to moderate acne and acne scars was conducted and subjects had split face treatment: 1 side with RFMN and the other side with bipolar RF. After 2 monthly treatments, results showed that RFMN was more effective in improving acne scars, and showed a reduction in acne lesions and sebum excretion.[7]

The results of an efficacy trial comparing RFMN with a 1550-nm Er:glass fractionated laser in the treatment of acne scars showed that both groups had statistically significant improvement compared with baseline. Although the laser group showed superior results, there was no significant difference between the 2 groups. However, more side effects were noted in the laser group (pain, erythema, edema, dryness), and other side effects, such as acne and PIH, were only reported in the laser group.[29]

## RADIOFREQUENCY MICRONEEDLING FOR SKIN REJUVENATION (LAXITY AND WRINKLES)

Another large area of interest in which RFMN is beginning to play a large role is in the improvement of skin laxity and texture through skin remodeling and collagen stimulation.

In a multicenter trial, the midface and lower face were treated with the Intensif device to assess lifting, tightening, and wrinkle reduction. Forty-nine subjects (skin types II–IV) received 3 monthly RFMN treatments on the cheeks, submandibular area, and the neck. Subject evaluation was done 3 months after the last treatment to assess lower face lifting and skin tightening. The Global Aesthetic Improvement Scale (GAIS) was used and results showed that 100% of subjects had improvement and 65% had significant improvement. For wrinkle reduction and improvement of skin texture, the Fitzpatrick Wrinkle and Elastosis Scale was used and results showed significant reduction from baseline (the average Fitzpatrick scores were 3.5 ± 1.66 at 3 months compared with 5.04 ± 1.22 at baseline).[30]

In another study, Lyons and colleagues[31] investigated the efficacy of RFMN for the improvement of wrinkles and skin laxity of the décolletage area. Twelve subjects received RFMN treatment every

ACTIVE ACNE

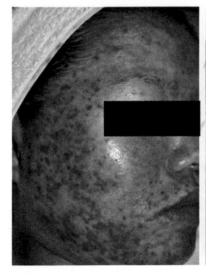 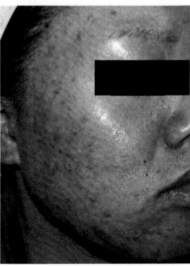

Before        After

**Fig. 2.** Before and 1 week after 2 INTRAcel treatments for active acne. (*Courtesy of* Jeisys Corporation, Seoul, KR; with permission.)

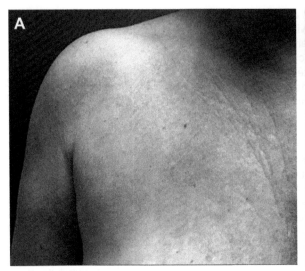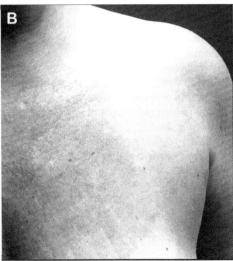

**Fig. 3.** (*A*) Before and (*B*) 30 days after 1 treatment with the Genius device for chest wrinkles. (*Courtesy of Lutronic Corporation, MA, USA; with permission.*)

3 weeks for a total of 3 treatments, using the Intensif device. One month following the last treatment was the evaluation using both the GAIS and patient-reported satisfaction. Results showed that 67% of subjects had at least a 1-point GAIS improvement and 80% of subjects were at least slightly satisfied[31] (**Fig. 3**).

A study done in Japan, in which 20 patients received 1 RFMN treatment to the face, showed that there was a significant volumetric reduction and skin tightening of the lower two-thirds of the face 6 months after the treatment when evaluated by three-dimensional volumetric assessment. Ninety-percent of patients were satisfied or very satisfied with the results.[32] Twelve months after the treatment, 15 of the study subjects were evaluated and showed significant volume reduction in the nasal and perioral area, proving the long-lasting effect of RFMN.[33]

When using RFMN for skin rejuvenation, studies reported a similar side effect profile to RFMN used for acne scars: transient erythema, edema, and pain.

Topical anesthesia is usually sufficient to prevent pain associated with the RFMN procedure. Most studies referenced in this article reported the use of topical anesthetic cream for 30 to 60 minutes before the procedure,[26–33] and 1 study[25] used topical anesthesia as well as nerve blocks.

## REFERENCES

1. Aust MC, Fernandes D, Kolokythas P, et al. Percutaneous collagen induction therapy: an alternative treatment for scars, wrinkles, and skin laxity. Plast Reconstr Surg 2008;121(4):1421–9.
2. Arnoczky SP, Aksan A. Thermal modification of connective tissues: basic science considerations and clinical implications. J Am Acad Orthop Surg 2000;8(5):305–13.
3. Zelickson BD, Kist D, Bernstein E, et al. Histological and ultrastructural evaluation of the effects of a radiofrequency-based nonablative dermal remodeling device: a pilot study. Arch Dermatol 2004;140(2):204–9.
4. Fitzpatrick R, Geronemus R, Goldberg D, et al. Multicenter study of noninvasive radiofrequency for periorbital tissue tightening. Lasers Surg Med 2003;33(4):232–42.
5. Alster TS, Tanzi E. Improvement of neck and cheek laxity with a nonablative radiofrequency device: a lifting experience. Dermatol Surg 2004;30:503–7.
6. Fritz M, Counters JT, Zelickson BD. Radiofrequency treatment for middle and lower face laxity. Arch Facial Plast Surg 2004;6(6):370–3.
7. Min S, Park SY, Yoon JY, et al. Comparison of fractional microneedling radiofrequency and bipolar radiofrequency on acne and acne scar and investigation of mechanism: comparative randomized controlled clinical trial. Arch Dermatol Res 2015;307(10):897–904.
8. Lee HS, Lee DH, Won CH, et al. Fractional rejuvenation using a novel bipolar radiofrequency system in Asian skin. Dermatol Surg 2011;37(11):1611–9.
9. Alster TS, Graham PM. Microneedling: a review and practical guide. Dermatol Surg 2018;44(3):397–404.
10. Fabbrocini G, Fardella N, Monfrecola A, et al. Acne scarring treatment using skin needling. Clin Exp Dermatol 2009;34(8):874–9.

11. Alam M, Han S, Pongprutthipan M, et al. Efficacy of a needling device for the treatment of acne scars: a randomized clinical trial. JAMA Dermatol 2014; 150(8):844–9.

12. Leheta TM, Abdel Hay RM, Hegazy RA, et al. Do combined alternating sessions of 1540 nm nonablative fractional laser and percutaneous collagen induction with trichloroacetic acid 20% show better results than each individual modality in the treatment of atrophic acne scars? A randomized controlled trial. J Dermatolog Treat 2014;25(2):137–41.

13. Cachafeiro T, Escobar G, Maldonado G, et al. Comparison of nonablative fractional erbium laser 1,340 nm and microneedling for the treatment of atrophic acne scars: a randomized clinical trial. Dermatol Surg 2016;42(2):232–41.

14. Fabbrocini G. Combined use of skin needling and platelet-rich plasma in acne scarring treatment. Cosmet Dermatol 2011;24(4):177–83.

15. Chawla S. Split face comparative study of microneedling with PRP Versus microneedling with vitamin C in treating atrophic post acne scars. J Cutan Aesthet Surg 2014;7(4):209–12.

16. Asif M, Kanodia S, Singh K. Combined autologous platelet-rich plasma with microneedling verses microneedling with distilled water in the treatment of atrophic acne scars: a concurrent split-face study. J Cosmet Dermatol 2016;15(4):434–43.

17. Dhurat R, Sukesh M, Avhad G, et al. A randomized evaluator blinded study of effect of microneedling in androgenetic alopecia: a pilot study. Int J Trichology 2013;5(1):6–11.

18. Fabbrocini G, De Vita V, Fardella N, et al. Skin needling to enhance depigmenting serum penetration in the treatment of melasma. Plast Surg Int 2011;2011:158241.

19. El-Domyati M, Barakat M, Awad S, et al. Multiple microneedling sessions for minimally invasive facial rejuvenation: an objective assessment. Int J Dermatol 2015;54(12):1361–9.

20. Ablon G. Safety and effectiveness of an automated microneedling device in improving the signs of aging skin. J Clin Aesthet Dermatol 2018;11(8):29–34.

21. Belenky I, Margulis A, Elman M, et al. Exploring channeling optimized radiofrequency energy: a review of radiofrequency history and applications in esthetic fields. Adv Ther 2012;29(3):249–66.

22. Lee SJ, Yeo UC, Wee SH, et al. Consensus recommendations on the use of a fractional radiofrequency microneedle and its applications in dermatologic laser surgery. Medical Lasers; Engineering, Basic Research, and Clinical Application 2014;3:5–10.

23. Hantash BM, Renton B, Berkowitz RL, et al. Pilot clinical study of a novel minimally invasive bipolar microneedle radiofrequency device. Lasers Surg Med 2009;41(2):87–95.

24. Hantash BM, Ubeid AA, Chang H, et al. Bipolar fractional radiofrequency treatment induces neoelastogenesis and neocollagenesis. Lasers Surg Med 2009;41(1):1–9.

25. Chandrashekar BS, Sriram R, Mysore R, et al. Evaluation of microneedling fractional radiofrequency device for treatment of acne scars. J Cutan Aesthet Surg 2014;7(2):93–7.

26. Pudukadan D. Treatment of acne scars on darker skin types using a noninsulated smooth motion, electronically controlled radiofrequency microneedles treatment system. Dermatol Surg 2017; 43(Suppl 1):S64–9.

27. Kim ST, Lee KH, Sim HJ, et al. Treatment of acne vulgaris with fractional radiofrequency microneedling. J Dermatol 2014;41(7):586–91.

28. Min S, Park SY, Yoon JY, et al. Fractional microneedling radiofrequency treatment for acne-related post-inflammatory erythema. Acta Derm Venereol 2016;96(1):87–91.

29. Chae WS, Seong JY, Jung HN, et al. Comparative study on efficacy and safety of 1550 nm Er:Glass fractional laser and fractional radiofrequency microneedle device for facial atrophic acne scar. J Cosmet Dermatol 2015;14(2):100–6.

30. Gold M, Taylor M, Rothaus K, et al. Non-insulated smooth motion, micro-needles RF fractional treatment for wrinkle reduction and lifting of the lower face: International study. Lasers Surg Med 2016; 48(8):727–33.

31. Lyons A, Roy J, Herrmann J, et al. Treatment of décolletage photoaging with fractional microneedling radiofrequency. J Drugs Dermatol 2018;17(1):74–6.

32. Tanaka Y. Long-term three-dimensional volumetric assessment of skin tightening using a sharply tapered non-insulated microneedle radiofrequency applicator with novel fractionated pulse mode in asians. Lasers Surg Med 2015;47(8):626–33.

33. Tanaka Y. Long-term nasal and peri-oral tightening by a single fractional noninsulated microneedle radiofrequency treatment. J Clin Aesthet Dermatol 2017;10(2):45–51.

# Microneedle Radiofrequency

Macrene Alexiades, MD, PhD[a,b],*

## KEYWORDS

- Microneedle • Radiofrequency • Skin laxity

## KEY POINTS

- Patient demand for nonsurgical alternatives to targeting skin laxity and rhytids have given rise to the advent of microneedle radiofrequency (RF), which provides direct *in situ* delivery, impedance measurements, temperature measurements, energy delivery controls, and targeting of various skin depths to achieve desired clinical outcomes.
- Microneedle RF is a breakthrough that controls penetration depth and delivery to specified temperatures and impedance measurements, which ensure significantly improved efficacy in the treatment of mild-to-moderate rhytids and skin laxity of the face, neck, and cellulite and laxity on other body sites.
- Combining microneedle RF with dermal fillers and neuromodulators may be used to further improve clinical outcomes and achieve high patient satisfaction.

## BACKGROUND

More than any other laser-based or energy-based technology, radiofrequency (RF) devices are the most used for the treatment of skin laxity. Skin laxity, manifested as sagging of the skin, is one of the primary findings in skin aging (**Table 1**). According to the survey by the American Society for Dermatologic Surgery, 67% of the population request treatment for sagging skin on the jawline and neck.[1] Although the gold standard for the treatment of facial and neck laxity is surgical rhytidectomy, there is high patient demand for nonsurgical alternatives that eliminate the need for systemic anesthesia, postsurgical morbidity, and the fear of altered cosmetic appearance. Nonsurgical skin-tightening technologies such as RF do not replace surgery for those with advanced to severe skin laxity, but key advances such as microneedle delivery provide clinically meaningful outcomes for those with mild-to-moderate skin laxity on the face and with cellulite or rhytids on the body, with minimal recovery and rare risk of side effects or complications.[2–4]

## CANDIDATE SELECTION

The ideal candidate for microneedle RF is one with mild-to-moderate skin laxity of the facial or neck skin or with cellulite or rhytids on the body. Chief complaints of patients with skin laxity include sagging, crepey, or loose skin on the face or neck, and deepening facial creases, jowls, lines, or folding on face and/or body. Patients with cellulite complain of linear undulations, dimples, or irregularity on the buttocks or thighs.

## DIAGNOSIS

A validated skin aging classification and grading scheme is presented with a verified scale for rhytides, laxity, and the subcategories of photoaging, including dyspigmentation, erythema/telangiectasia, solar elastosis, keratosis, and textural changes (see **Table 1**).[5,6] The clinical signs of skin laxity of the face include nasolabial folds, melolabial folds, jowls, submental and submandibular redundancy, and neck platysmal strands. Loss of elasticity and recoil are clinical findings.

[a] Yale University School of Medicine, New Haven, CT, USA; [b] University of Athens Sygros Hospital, Athens, Greece
* Dermatology and Laser Surgery Center of New York, 955 Park Avenue, New York, NY 10028.
*E-mail address:* email@nyderm.org

Facial Plast Surg Clin N Am 28 (2020) 9–15
https://doi.org/10.1016/j.fsc.2019.09.013
1064-7406/20/© 2019 Elsevier Inc. All rights reserved.

**Table 1**
Quantitative comprehensive grading scale of rhytides, laxity, and photoaging

| | | Alexiades Classification and Grading Scale of Skin Aging | | | | | | |
|---|---|---|---|---|---|---|---|---|
| Grade | Descriptive Parameter | Rhytides | Laxity | Elastosis | Dyschromia | Erythema-Telangiectasia (E-T) | Keratoses | Texture |
| 0 | None | None | None | None | None | None | None | None |
| 1 | Mild | Wrinkles in motion, few, superficial | Localized to nasolabial (nl) folds | Early, minimal yellow hue | Few (1–3) discrete small (<5 mm) lentigines | Pink E or few T, localized to single site | Few | Subtle irregularity |
| 1.5 | Mild | Wrinkles in motion, multiple, superficial | Localized, nl and early melolabial (ml) folds | Yellow hue or early, localized periorbital (po) elastotic beads (eb) | Several (3–6) discrete small lentigines | Pink E or several T, localized to 2 sites | Several | Mild irregularity in few areas |
| 2 | Moderate | Wrinkles at rest, few, localized, superficial | Localized, nl/ml folds, early jowls, early submental/submandibular (sm) | Yellow hue, localized po eb | Multiple (7–10) small lentigines | Red E or multiple T, localized to 2 sites | Multiple, small | Rough in few localized sites |
| 2.5 | Moderate | Wrinkles at rest, multiple, localized, superficial | Localized, prominent nl/ml folds, jowls and sm | Yellow hue, po and malar eb | Multiple small and few large lentigines | Red E or multiple T, localized to 3 sites | Multiple, large | Rough in several localized areas |
| 3 | Advanced | Wrinkles at rest, multiple, forehead, periorbital and perioral sites, superficial | Prominent nl/ml folds, jowls and sm. Early neck strands | Yellow hue, eb involving po, malar, and other sites | Many (10–20) small and large lentigines | Violaceous E or many T, multiple sites | Many | Rough in multiple localized sites |
| 3.5 | Advanced | Wrinkles at rest, multiple, generalized, superficial; few, deep | Deep nl/ml folds, prominent jowls and sm, prominent neck strands | Deep yellow hue, extensive eb with little uninvolved skin | Numerous (>20) or multiple large lentigines with little uninvolved skin | Violaceous E, numerous T, little uninvolved skin | Little uninvolved skin | Mostly rough, little uninvolved skin |
| 4 | Severe | Wrinkles throughout, numerous, extensively distributed, deep | Marked nl/ml folds, jowls and sm, neck redundancy and strands | Deep yellow hue, eb throughout, comedones | Numerous lentigines, extensive, no uninvolved skin | Deep, violaceous E, numerous T throughout | No uninvolved skin | Rough throughout |

This 4-point grading scale has been extensively tested and used for evaluating laser-based and energy-based cosmetic treatments.
*Data from* Refs.[2–6]

Although body skin laxity lacks a validated grading scale, the relative firmness of body skin has been assessed by the presence or absence of surface irregularities.[2–6] Skin laxity on the body similarly presents with rhytids, lack of recoil, folds upon flexion, linear undulations, and poor texture. Cellulite grading scales have been variably tested and used.[4]

## PATHOGENESIS

The dermal matrix of connective tissue confers the properties of elasticity, recoil, and tensile strength. The properties of elasticity and resilience are attributed to the elastic fiber system, which confers the deformability and passive recoil of tissue. Collagen fibers provide tensile strength while hyaluronic acid provides turgor and skin moisture. In diseases characterized by alterations in elastic fibers, the skin is loose and sagging with a loss of recoil, elasticity, and resilience.[6–10] Elastic fiber mutations, deficiency, degradation, or alteration result in reduced skin elasticity and increased skin laxity, which may be reversed through stimulation of neoelastogenesis.[6–10] By contrast, loss of collagen is more closely associated with rhytid formation. During the aging process, collagen and elastin synthesis decrease, and elastin fibers are degraded through sun exposure starting in the third decade of life.

Heat denaturation of collagen and dermal structures has been shown to induce histologic dermal remodeling and clinical laxity reduction.[11] In work by the author, it was discovered that collagen greater than 70°C, which results in fully denatured collagen, is associated with poorer clinical outcomes; in contrast, intradermal temperatures of 62°C to 67°C, which are associated with partially denatured collagen, result in superior clinical efficacy in rhytid and laxity reduction. The author has thus theorized that heat-induced partially denatured collagens reveal RGD sequences that via a signaling cascade result in induction of neocollagenesis and neoelastogenesis.[11] The neocollagenesis process has been demonstrated to take up to 12 months following treatment and correlates with progressive clinical improvement.

## MECHANISM OF ACTION

RF delivery to the skin creates thermal, mechanical, and biochemical effects that induce dermal remodeling. The increases in collagen, elastin, and hyaluronic acid increase volume and improve the elastic properties of the skin.[12,13] RF delivers controlled thermal injury that induces neocollagenesis and neoelastogenesis, which correlate with clinical rhytid and laxity reduction.

RF is in the 3-kHz to 24-GHz frequency range and, when delivered as an oscillating electrical current, it induces collisions between charged atoms and molecules in tissue, generating heat.[14] The penetration depth of RF is inversely proportional to frequency; lower RF frequencies penetrate more deeply when applied to the skin surface. Heat is generated from the resistance of tissue components to the movement of charged and polar molecules within the oscillating RF field. This resistance, termed impedance, generates heat relative to the amount of current and time, converting electrical current to thermal energy.

## SUBTYPES

RF devices may be classified as noninvasive and minimally invasive, the latter being delivered by microneedles or probes. RF may be classified according to electrode configuration: monopolar RF uses a single electrode and a grounding pad; unipolar RF is via antenna transmission; bipolar and tripolar RF use multiple electrodes in the handpiece tip whereby the current traverses the skin via a closed circuit. The penetration depth of multipolar RF when delivered on the skin surface is approximately one-half the distance between the electrodes. Microneedle RF delivery bypasses these barriers and delivers energy directly into the dermis and subcutis. The singular breakthrough of the first microneedle RF device (Profound; Candela Medical, Wayland, MA) is that it uses thermistors in the electrode needle tips, allowing real-time feedback of both impedance and temperature.[2–4,13]

The penetration depth depends on delivery mode (skin surface, needle-based, or probe-based), electrode configuration (monopolar or multipolar), tissue type (skin, fat), and the frequency of the current. Structures with higher conductivity and impedance generate more heat: fat, bone, and dry skin have low conductivities such that current flows around rather than through these structures; hydrated skin possesses high electrical conductivity via the effects of water dipole moment, thus allowing greater penetration of current. Improved results are observed with coupling fluid.

### Monopolar Radiofrequency

Clinical study results from monopolar RF treatment were first reported in 2003 by the author's group for the jowls and neck, and by Fitzpatrick and colleagues for the periorbital area.[14,15] The original single-pass, high-energy method was later compared with the low-energy, multiple-pass technique demonstrating response rates of 54% and 92%, respectively, at 6 months. Anesthesia is no longer required and adverse events were also reduced to less than 0.05% with the modified protocol.[11] The device does not provide real-time temperature feedback, so reliance on patient verbal feedback regarding heat pain is still required.

An alternative skin surface applied monopolar RF device operating at a frequency of 1 and 2 MHz, electrode sizes of 16, 25, and 40 cm$^2$, and providing skin surface temperature feedback was developed to treat skin laxity (truSculpt; Cutera, Brisbane, CA). The author determined that skin surface temperatures of 42°C to 46°C are necessary to attain tissue tightening. Whereas the 1-MHz and 16-cm$^2$ tip is used for skin laxity, the recent 2-MHz (truSculpt 3D; Cutera) large handpieces target skin laxity and fat reduction, with approximately 25% circumferential reduction in more than 90% of patients.[16]

Another skin surface–applied monopolar RF device (Pelleve; Ellman, Oceanside, NY) operates at 4 MHz with handpiece tip sizes from 7.5 to 20 mm$^2$. Fifty percent skin laxity and textural improvement was reported at 1 year following 6 treatments.[17]

### Probe-delivered monopolar radiofrequency
Monopolar RF may be delivered via a probe to the subdermal plane for skin tightening of the jawline and neck (ThermiTight; ThermiAesthetics, Irving, TX). A blunt 10-cm, 18-gauge percutaneous treatment probe is inserted subdermally; the distal end administers the current and contains a temperature sensor that initiates an automatic feedback loop to maintain subdermal tissue temperature set at 50°C to 60°C. Subdermal temperatures of 65°C and 50°C were found to correlate with skin surface temperatures of 41.6°C and 41.1°C, respectively.[18,19]

### Microneedle-delivered monopolar radiofrequency
A variation on monopolar RF may be delivered via uninsulated microneedle electrodes that are grounded to the pad in the handpiece tip to create a closed loop (VoluDerm, Pollogen; Lumenis, Santa Clara, CA). The RF current is delivered via a tip composed of an array of 36 microneedles that penetrate the treated area as the needle temperature increases, resulting in a treatment that does not require topical or local anesthesia. The full-length heating of the needles results in heating of both dermal and epidermal layers while superficially penetrating the dermis (M.A., in preparation).

### Unipolar Radiofrequency
In 2008, the author invented the mobile delivery method with a combined unipolar/bipolar RF device.[20] Mobile delivery was used to increase fluence delivery to dermis while allowing cooling of the epidermis. Mild efficacy in skin tightening was observed in a split-face controlled trial comparing the unipolar with the bipolar RF handpiece. Skin surface temperature profiles of 40°C to 43°C were required, but efficacy was limited. The same group reported efficacy in skin tightening on the body using a similar mobile protocol.[21]

### Bipolar Radiofrequency

#### Skin surface bipolar radiofrequency
Many skin surface–applied bipolar RF skin-tightening devices have been developed that combine light energy or vacuum (Galaxy, Aurora, Polaris, ReFirme, Sublime, and Vela III systems: Syneron Candela, Wayland, MA; Aluma: Lumenis). RF current flows between the electrodes in the handpiece tip via a closed loop through the skin but is limited with respect to penetration depth. Arcing and burns may occur when inadequate coupling gel is applied and the handpiece makes incomplete contact with the skin. Modest efficacy has been demonstrated in clinical studies with skin surface RF.[22–26]

**Needle-delivered bipolar radiofrequency** Over the course of the last decade, the author and others have pioneered needle-delivered bipolar RF (Profound; Syneron Candela). The first device to deliver RF via a microneedle electrode array directly into the reticular dermis, bypassing the epidermis and papillary dermis, provided the first *in situ* real-time impedance and temperature feedback using thermistors in the electrode tips (**Fig. 1**). This device has undergone repeated improvements over the years in needle configuration,

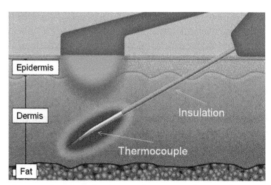

**Fig. 1.** Microneedle RF handpiece configuration.

gauge, manufacturing, and refinements in the protocol to optimize clinical outcomes. Single-use treatment cartridges deliver 5 pairs of independently controlled, 32-gauge, bipolar 250-μm microneedles spaced 1.25 mm apart; each needle pair is independently sensed and powered by the RF generator. The proximal 3 mm of the 6-mm needle is insulated to protect the superficial portion of the skin during treatment while the distal 3-mm length is exposed to allow electrical current flow between needle pairs to generate 3-dimensional zones of thermal effects in the target. The dermal handpiece is at a 25° angle so that the tips of the needles are at a 2-mm depth from the epidermis. As current flows between each needle pair, fractionated zones (one between each pair) of thermal injury are situated in the dermis 2 mm from the surface of the skin. Epidermal cooling is achieved via an integrated thermokinetic cooling bar on the applicator. Intradermal targeting is ensured by impedance measurements in the needle tips and software, ensuring firing within a specified impedance range. A target temperature is selected by the user and energy is delivered until the target temperature is attained and energy titrated to maintain precise target temperature for a selected pulse duration. The subcutaneous handpiece delivers bipolar RF pulses using 5 pairs of microneedle electrodes deployed into the dermis at an angle of 75° with the exposed portion extending from 3.9 to 5.8 mm beneath the skin surface (Profound Sub-Q; Syneron Candela). Zones of thermal injury with real-time temperature monitoring using temperature sensors in each electrode tip maintain a preselected target temperature regardless of varying skin conditions and improve consistency between patients.

The author's group compared baseline and 3- to 6-month follow-up photographs of 15 patients who underwent skin tightening using a microneedle RF device with those of 6 patients who had undergone rhytidectomy.[2] The RF-device patients were judged to have a 16% improvement from baseline and the surgical patients were judged to have a 49% improvement from baseline laxity grades, or a 0.46 versus 1.20 laxity grade reduction, respectively. The laxity grade reduction result from a single microneedle RF treatment was 37% that of a surgical facelift.[2] In the subsequent multicenter clinical trial and multiarm studies of target dermal temperatures ranging from 52°C to 78°C, the author and colleagues discovered that temperature of 67°C in their cohort resulted in maximal neocollagenesis, neoelastogenesis, and hyaluronic acid production, and correlated clinically with maximal rhytid and laxity reduction and a 100% response rate.[3] Higher and lower target temperatures demonstrated less efficacy. The findings using needle-delivered RF support the theory that partially denatured collagen is more effective at triggering a strong wound-healing response.[3] **Fig. 2** shows 2 sets of "before" and "after" photographs following a single microneedle RF treatment (Profound, Candela). Arrows indicate findings of laxity at baseline including jowls and submental laxity at baseline, and significant reduction of jowls and submental laxity with restoration of mandibular definition on follow-up after a single treatment. Similar skin-tightening effects were observed on body skin laxity when the subcutaneous handpiece was used to treat cellulite.[4] When treating with microneedle RF on the body skin, a reduction in linear undulations and textural irregularities was observed.

Numerous needle-delivered bipolar RF devices have been developed. One device allows for adjustable needle depths to 0.5, 1.0, 1.5, 2.0 and 3.5 mm (Infini; Lutronic, Billerica, MA). The device offers a 49-needle tip (10 mm × 10 mm, 7 × 7 needles) and a 16-needle tip (5 mm × 5 mm, 4 × 4 needles). The microneedles are surgical stainless-steel gold-coated for conductivity and then double coated with an insulating silicon compound, except for the distal 300-μm tip. The needles have a diameter of 200 μm and point diameter of 20 μm. The

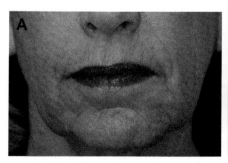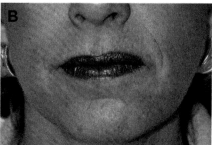

**Fig. 2.** Microneedle RF clinical outcomes showing 2 sets of before (A) and after (B) photographs following a single microneedle RF treatment (Profound, Candela).

insulation restricts the active area of the micro-needle electrodes to the tip, and there is no electrothermal damage delivered to the epidermis. Clinical trials have demonstrated wrinkle reduction following treatment with this device, with clinician-assessed overall efficacy and patient satisfaction index similar at from 80.7% to 88.9% and 81.3% to 85.9%.[27] Although the system lacks real-time temperature feedback, a recent improvement has incorporated impedance measurements (Genius, Lutronic).

Another bipolar microneedle RF device (Intensif; EndyMed Medical, Caesarea, Israel) includes 25 noninsulated gold-plated microneedle electrodes 300 μm in diameter at the base, gradually tapering to a sharp edge.[28] Penetration depth of up to 3.5 mm may be administered at 0.1-mm digitally controlled increments. Maximal power is 25 W with a maximal pulse duration of 200 - milliseconds. The electrical impedance difference between the epidermis (high) and the dermis (low) ensures RF flow through the dermis. The RF emission delivered throughout the length of the needle results in effective coagulation with minimal or no bleeding, and dermal heating.[28]

Another microneedle bipolar RF device (Fractora; Invasix, Lake Forest, CA) administers 1 MHz to RF-conducting needles, alternating current with 2 long side electrodes. The handpiece cartridges come as 600-μm or 3000-μm long needles, which are 200 × 300 μm wide at the base, for mid-dermal and deep dermal or subdermal delivery, respectively.[29] The mid-dermal delivers 60 microneedles while the full dermal or deep dermal/subdermal handpiece contains 24 uncoated or coated needles, respectively. The handpiece is loaded to the Fractora platform (also applicable to InMode or BodyTite platforms; Invasix/InMode MD, Israel). The device has been reported to result in significant improvement in acne and acne scars.[29]

## SUMMARY

Patient demand for nonsurgical alternatives to targeting skin laxity and rhytids have given rise to the advent of microneedle RF, which provides direct *in situ* delivery, impedance measurements, temperature measurements, energy delivery controls, and targeting of various skin depths to achieve desired clinical outcomes. Microneedle RF is a breakthrough that controls penetration depth and delivery to specified temperatures and impedance measurements, which ensure significantly improved efficacy in the treatment of mild-to-moderate rhytids and skin laxity of the face and neck, and cellulite and laxity on other body sites. Although surgical face lifting remains the gold standard, microneedle RF provides a clinically meaningful alternative for those who wish to avoid surgery or who have a milder condition. Combining microneedle RF with dermal fillers and neuromodulators may be used to further improve clinical outcomes and achieve high patient satisfaction.

## DISCLOSURE

Dr. Alexiades serves on the Medical Advisory Board of Candela and has received research grants from Candela, Cutera, Allergan, and Biofrontera.

## REFERENCES

1. American Society for Dermatologic Surgery (ASDS) 2015 Consumer Survey on cosmetic dermatologic procedures. Data were collected from 7,315 consumers through a blind online survey in spring 2015. Available at: https://www.asds.net/Portals/0/PDF/consumer-survey-2015-infographic.pdf.
2. Alexiades-Armenakas M, Rosenberg D, Renton B, et al. Blinded, randomized quantitative grading comparison of minimally-invasive fractional radiofrequency and surgical facelift for the treatment of skin laxity. Arch Dermatol 2010;146(4):396–405.
3. Alexiades-Armenakas M, Sarnoff D, Gotkin R, et al. Multi-center clinical study and review of fractional ablative co2 laser resurfacing for the treatment of rhytides, photoaging, scars and striae. J Drugs Dermatol 2011;10(4):352–62.
4. Alexiades M, Munavalli G, Goldberg D, et al. Prospective multicenter clinical trial of a temperature-controlled subcutaneous microneedle fractional bipolar RF system for the treatment of cellulite. Dermatol Surg 2018;44(10):1262–71.
5. Alexiades-Armenakas M. A quantitative and comprehensive grading scale for rhytides, laxity and photoaging. J Drugs Dermatol 2006;5(8):808–9.
6. Alexiades-Armenakas MR, Dover JS, Arndt KA. The spectrum of laser skin resurfacing: non-ablative, fractional and ablative laser resurfacing. J Am Acad Dermatol 2008;58(5):719–37 [quiz: 738–40].
7. El-Domyati M, Attia S, Saleh F, et al. Intrinsic aging vs. photoaging: a comparative histopathological, immunohistochemical, and ultrastructural study of skin. Exp Dermatol 2002;11:398–405.
8. Kielty CM, Sherratt MJ, Shuttleworth CA. Elastic fibres. J Cell Sci 2002;115:2817–28.
9. Lewis KG, Bercovitch L, Dill SW, et al. Acquired disorders of elastic tissue: part I. Increased elastic tissue and solar elastotic syndromes. J Am Acad Dermatol 2004;51:1–21.

10. Lewis KG, Bercovitch L, Dill SW, et al. Acquired disorders of elastic tissue: part II. decreased elastic tissue. J Am Acad Dermatol 2004;51:165–85.

11. Alexiades M, Berube D. Randomized, blinded, 3-arm clinical trial assessing optimal temperature and duration for treatment with minimally invasive fractional RF. Dermatol Surg 2015;41(5):623–32.

12. Alexiades-Armenakas M. Aging facial skin: infrared broad band light technologies. Facial Plast Surg Clin North Am 2011;19(2):361–70.

13. Willey A, Kilmer S, Newman J, et al. Elastometry and clinical results after bipolar radiofrequency treatment of skin. Dermatol Surg 2010;36(6):877–84.

14. Jacobson LG, Alexiades-Armenakas MR, Bernstein L, et al. Treatment of nasolabial folds and jowls with a non-invasive RF device. Arch Dermatol 2003;139(10):1313–20.

15. Fitzpatrick R, Geronemus R, Goldberg D, et al. Multicenter study of noninvasive RF for periorbital tissue tightening. Lasers Surg Med 2003;33:232–42.

16. Sugawara J, Kou S, Kokubo K, et al. Application for lower facial fat reduction and tightening by static type monopolar 1-MHz radio frequency for body contouring. Lasers Surg Med 2017;49(8):750–5.

17. Taub AF, Tucker RD, Palange A. Facial tightening with an advanced 4-MHz monopolar RF device. J Drugs Dermatol 2012;11(11):1288–94.

18. Key DJ. Integration of thermal imaging with subsurface RF thermistor heating for the purpose of skin tightening and contour improvement: a retrospective review of clinical efficacy. J Drugs Dermatol 2014; 13(12):1485–9.

19. Friedman DJ, Gilead LT. The use of hybrid RF device for the treatment of rhytides and lax skin. Dermatol Surg 2007;33:543–55.

20. Alexiades-Armenakas MR, Dover JS, Arndt KA. Unipolar vs. bipolar RF treatment of rhytides and laxity using a mobile painless delivery method. Lasers Surg Med 2008;40(7):446–53.

21. Alexiades-Armenakas MR, Dover JS, Arndt KA. Unipolar RF treatment to improve the appearance of cellulite. J Cosmet Laser Ther 2008;10(3): 148–53.

22. Doshi SN, Alster TS. Combined diode laser and RF energy for rhytides and skin laxity: investigation of a novel device. J Cosmet Laser Ther 2005;7:11–5.

23. Sadick NS, Alexiades-Armenakas M, Bitter P Jr, et al. Enhanced full-face skin rejuvenation using synchronous intense pulsed optical and conducted bipolar RF energy (ELOS): introducing selective radiophotothermolysis. J Eur Acad Dermatol Venereol 2005;4:181–6.

24. Alexiades-Armenakas M. Rhytides, laxity, and photoaging treated with a combination of RF, diode laser, and pulsed light and assessed with a comprehensive grading scale. J Drugs Dermatol 2006;5(8): 731–8.

25. Yu CS, Yeung CK, Shek SY, et al. Combined infrared light and bipolar RF for skin tightening in Asians. Lasers Surg Med 2007;39(6):471–5.

26. Gold MH, Goldman MP, Rao J, et al. Treatment of wrinkles and elastosis using vacuum-assisted bipolar RF heating of the dermis. Dermatol Surg 2007;33: 300–9.

27. Calderhead RG, Goo BL, Lauro F, et al. The clinical efficacy and safety of microneedling fractional RF in the treatment of facial wrinkles: a multicenter study with the infini system in 499 patients 2013. white paper. Available at: us.aesthetic.lutronic.com.

28. Gold M, Taylor M, Rothaus K, et al. Non-insulated smooth motion, micro-needles RF. Lasers Surg Med 2016;48(8):727–33.

29. Dayan E, Chia C, Burns AJ, Theodorou S. Adjustable depth fractional radiofrequency combined with bipolar radiofrequency: a minimally invasive combination treatment for skin laxity. Aesthet Surg J 2019;39(Supplement_3):S112–9.

# New Developments for Fractional Co$_2$ Resurfacing for Skin Rejuvenation and Scar Reduction

Matteo Tretti Clementoni, MD[a],*, Valerio Pedrelli, MD[a],
Giovanna Zaccaria, MD[a], Paolo Pontini, MD[a], Laura Romana Motta, MD[a],
Ernest A. Azzopardi, MD, MSc Surg PhD, MRCSEd, MRCSEng (Ad Eudem), Dip spec laser, FRSB, FRCSEd (Plast)[a,b]

## KEYWORDS

- Fractional Co$_2$ • Resurfacing • Laser-assisted drug delivery • Scars

## KEY POINTS

- Fractional Co$_2$ resurfacing offers a very good outcome with a short downtime and a very high safety profile.
- Best rejuvenation outcomes can be achieved when the procedure is customized on each patient affecting different layers of the skin.
- Fractional Co$_2$ can determine a significant change in dermal architecture of severe burn scars, improving function and appearance of burn patients.
- The laser-assisted drug delivery induces a great and uniform absorption of drugs inside the skin.

## INTRODUCTION: THREE SIGNIFICANT DEVELOPMENTS IN RECENT YEARS

The drive to attain cosmetic facial improvement with rapid recovery and minimal risk has galvanized laser treatments. The introduction, 15 years ago, of nonablative fractional devices and of ablative fractional devices immediately thereafter, provided laser specialists with the potential for a safe and significantly effective cosmetic outcome. A few years later, the realisation that the same devices can safely and effectively improve function and appearance of severe burn scars, produced a step-change in management of secondary burn reconstruction. The possibility of adding laser treatments to the classical surgical approaches in restoring function and appearance of severe burn patients gave the opportunity to the laser operators to effectively improve the quality of life of patients presenting this kind of severe scars. Finally, use of ablative fractional lasers to faciltiate trans-dermal drug delivery (laser-assisted drug delivery, or LADD) opened up a new dimension in personalised medicine, and precision therapeutics. This laser-assisted drug delivery allows physicians to deliver drugs, such as triamcinolone, 5-fluorouracil, botulinum toxin, and poly-l-lactic acid (PLLA), at a precise depth inside the skin. These 3 developments have a common denominator: the principle of the customization of the procedure. The next paragraphs describe how the authors use an ultrapulse Co$_2$, customizing the procedures to each patient and the principles and the rationale behind them.

### The Device and the Settings

The authors use a radiofrequency excited ultrapulse Co$_2$ laser (Ultrapulse Encore; - Lumenis

Ernest Azzopardi's research is currently supported by the Dowager Eleanor Peel Foundation Trust.
[a] Laserplast SrL StP, Piazza Eleonora Duse 2 Milano, Republic of Italy; [b] R&D Department, Swansea Bay University Health Board and the Welsh Centre for Burns and Plastic Surgery, Moriston Hospital, Swansea SA6 6NL, United Kingdom
* Corresponding author.
E-mail address: mtretti@laserplast.org

Facial Plast Surg Clin N Am 28 (2020) 17–28
https://doi.org/10.1016/j.fsc.2019.09.002
1064-7406/20/© 2019 Elsevier Inc. All rights reserved.

facialplastic.theclinics.com

Ltd, Yokneam, Israel) with a pulse duration around 500 microseconds. It can deliver 225 mJ of energy having 240 W of power to tissue. The decision to use an ultrapulse $CO_2$ depends on the features this device offers in the interaction laser/tissue. With a short-pulse duration, the collateral thermal damage is minimal and the downtime is very short. The ablation threshold of an ultrapulse $CO_2$ is 3 times lower than a continuous wave (CW) $CO_2$ (which means that 3 times less energy must be applied to start to ablate skin). In a hypothetical comparison between an ultrapulse $CO_2$ and a CW device (where the pulse duration is longer than 2 microseconds), it can be demonstrated that if the same spot size and the same energy with the ultrapulse $CO_2$ are used, the ablation channel will be deeper, the ablated volume will be larger, and the collateral thermal damage will be lower[1,2] (**Fig. 1**).

The device has 2 hand pieces. One hand piece is called CPG (computer pattern generator) and creates ablation of 1300 microns of diameter, whereas the second is a microscanner that creates ablation of only 120 microns of diameter. CPG settings are described by energy (mJ), frequency (Hz), and 3 numbers: the first indicates the shape pattern (line, hexagon, square, and so forth); the second indicates the shape dimension (the higher the number, the higher the dimension), while the third indicates the microshots density. The microscanner settings are described by energy (mJ), frequency (Hz), and, as before, shape, dimension, and density of the microshots.

### Fractional Skin Resurfacing for Rejuvenation: The Multilayer Technique

Aging skin processes are complex and include bone resorption, fat resorption, soft tissue ptosis

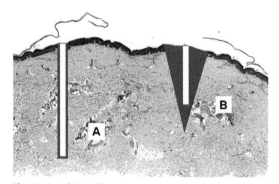

**Fig. 1.** Applying the same energy on the same spot size, a $CO_2$ laser with a short-pulse duration (*A*) will determine a deeper penetration, a large volume ablation, and (*B*) less thermal damage than a $CO_2$ laser with a long-pulse duration.

for ligament, and skin laxity and superficial damage owing to the UV irradiation. Although volume and shape of soft tissues of the face can only minimally be affected by a $CO_2$ fractional resurfacing, superficial photodamage can be effectively treated. The superficial photodamage consists of wrinkles, lentigines, sun spots, and a wide suggestion of yellowness and grayness of the skin. In a schematic way and using a sketch, the photodamage can be represented as in **Fig. 2**.

The customized plan is obtained by marking all the wrinkles and the biggest lentigines (**Fig. 3**) with a skin marker. A numbing cream (7% lidocaine–7% tetracaine) is applied on the skin for 1 hour (Pliaglis; Galderma, Uppsala, Sweden) and then carefully removed with dry gauze. A nonalcoholic disinfectant is then passed on the skin without removing the marks. The procedure is then performed with the help of a device that emits cold air (−20°C; Cryo 6; Zimmer, Neu-Ulm, Germany) to make it more comfortable for the patient (see **Fig. 3**).

### THE TECHNIQUE

The multilayer technique can be divided into 5 steps:

1. Step 1: Use the microscanner hand piece. Using a short linear shape, the authors follow each wrinkle, trying to hit the base of it. They use 15 to 40 mJ depending on the skin thickness (the thicker the skin, the higher the energy) and a density of 10%. The frequency is always 300 Hz. The aim of this pass is to deliver a large amount of heat at the base of each wrinkle to obtain an important new collagen production exactly where needed (**Fig. 4**).
2. Step 2: Again use the microscanner hand piece. Using a rectangular shape, the authors decrease the energy (15–25 mJ), but they increase the density to 15% to 20%. As before, the authors follow the route of each wrinkle (**Fig. 5**). The aim of this pass is to obtain shrinkage of the wrinkle. If they have wrinkles very close to each other, the authors use a square shape, and with the same settings of energy and density, they cover all the affected area.

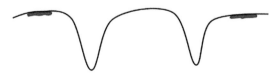

**Fig. 2.** The 2 major features of aging skin: wrinkles and lentigines.

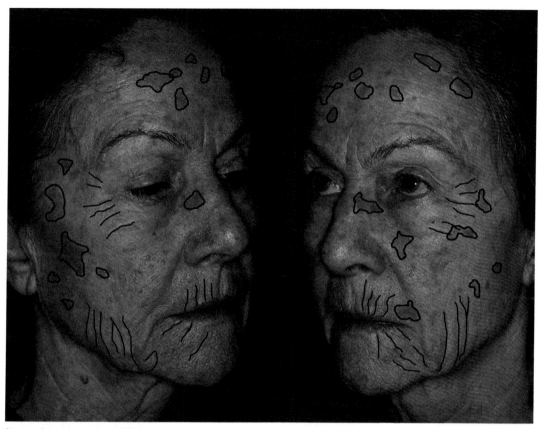

**Fig. 3.** The preoperative marking.

3. Step 3: Again, using the microscanner hand piece and using a square shape with a medium amount of energy and density (15–20 mJ and 10%–15% of density), the authors treat both cheeks. The aim of this pass is to obtain a tightening effect of the areas where the laxity of soft tissues is more visible (**Fig. 6**).

4. Step 4: Using the CPG scanner and using a circular shape, the authors remove all lentigines and pigmented lesions. They use very low energy (30–40 mJ) but very high frequency (350 Hz) and very high density (density 9). This way the authors are not doing a "fractionated procedure," but they are trying to ablate all pigmented lesions using a nonpigmented specific device. These pure ablative settings (very low energy with high frequency and high density)

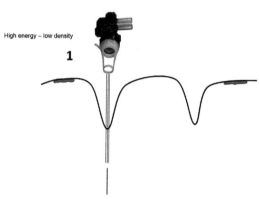

**Fig. 4.** Step 1 of the multilayer technique.

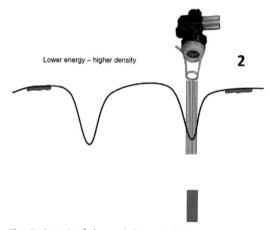

**Fig. 5.** Step 2 of the multilayer technique.

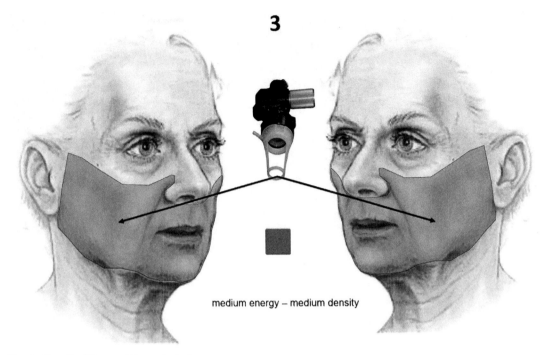

medium energy – medium density

**Fig. 6.** Step 3 of the multilayer technique.

allow the authors to ablate the lesions, delivering as little heat as possible[3] (**Fig. 7**).

5. Step 5: The last pass is performed using the CPG hand piece. The authors use a large hexagonal shape with 125 to 150 mJ of energy, 125 to 150 Hz of frequency, and density of 3 (covering this way 82% of the surface) (**Fig. 8**). They cover the full face, and for 1 cm below the jaw line, the authors reduce the energy to 70 to 80 mJ. These different settings are to attempt to feather the result, to avoid visualizing a clear, sharp line between the treated and nontreated areas. The same results can be obtained simply by inclining the hand piece at 45° and transforming the microshot from circular to oval.

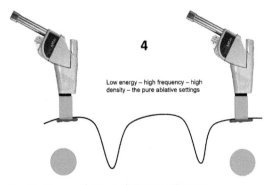

Low energy – high frequency – high density – the pure ablative settings

**Fig. 7.** Step 4 of the multilayer technique.

## PRETREATMENT AND POSTTREATMENT REGIMEN

The authors exclude patients from the treatment who present the following: (i) pregnancy; (ii) lactation; (iii) history of keloids; (iv) history of severe herpes infections; (v) likelihood of poor compliance; (vi) presence of an active infectious disease or other inflammatory or neoplastic skin diseases; (vii) psychiatric diseases; and (viii) unrealistic expectations. Starting the night before the treatment, all patients were treated with oral cefixime (400 mg every day for 5 days), valacyclovir (1000 mg, 2 every day for 14 days), and fluconazole (100 mg /day for 8 days). Patients with dark skin type or patients prone to a postinflammatory hyperpigmentation are treated for 5 weeks before the treatment with modified Kligman-Willis formula (tretinoin, hydroquinone, vitamin C and hydrocortisone in a water-based cream). These small fine crusts must not be removed because they can be used as a completely biocompatible wound dressing. Just after the end of the procedure, wet cold gauzes are applied to the treated surface, kept moist and cool using cold saline solution. Twenty to 30 minutes after the treatment or when the pain or burning sensation eased off, a thin layer of an ointment (Aquaphor; Eucerin, Collegno, Italy) was applied. Cleansing was allowed only with a gentle cleanser starting from 36 hours after the treatment. Before leaving the office, all patients

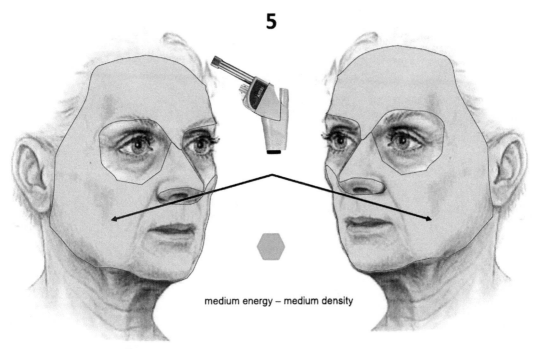

medium energy – medium density

**Fig. 8.** Step 5 of the multilayer technique.

are instructed to repeatedly apply the ointment for the next 3 to 5 days and are advised against picking or scrubbing the skin. All patients are also strictly instructed to repeatedly apply topical sunblock preparations for 60 days starting on the day of the disappearance of the small crusts. The authors also ask patients not to go directly into the sun (beach vacation or mountain vacation) for 2 months after the procedure. The downtime (calculated as the time needed for the crusts to disappear) is usually 5 to 7 days. After this interval of time, the patient will present a uniform erythema that will disappear in a couple of weeks. Patients with dark skin or patients prone to develop postinflammatory hyperpigmentation will start to apply the Kligman-Willis modified formula (previously described) for 6 to 8 weeks.

## RESULTS

The degree of photoaging and the efficacy of the treatment can be evaluated using a 5-point scale based on the suggestion of Dover and colleagues.[4] A global score can be recorded as well as that of 5 photodamage variables: fine lines, mottled pigmentation, sallow complexion, tactile roughness, and coarse wrinkles. Based on this 5-point scale, the authors demonstrated[5,6] that the technique with the customization of the procedure offers very good outcomes (**Fig. 9**) and that the results can be considered stable 24 months after the procedure (**Fig. 10**).

The adverse events are usually rare and transitory (the authors observed only a few cases of prolonged erythema and hyperpigmentations, which disappeared spontaneously in a maximum of 4 weeks). Severe adverse events, such as scars, infections, or hypopigmentations, have never been observed.

## AN OVERVIEW ON THE SCIENCE BEHIND THE ULTRAPULSE FRACTIONAL $CO_2$ PROCEDURE ON SEVERE BURN SCARS

The exact mechanism of action at the base of the outcomes that can be observed after an ultrapulse fractional $CO_2$ procedure has yet to be fully understood. Creating thousands of thin, deep holes inside the burn scar, 2 immediate mechanical results can be achieved. With a spot size of 120 µm and a maximum energy of 150 mJ, the SCAARFX mode (synergistic coagulation and ablation for advanced resurfacing) allows attainment of a penetration depth of 4.5 mm. The SCAARFX mode (synergistic coagulation and ablation for advanced resurfacing) allows attainment of a penetration depth of 4.5mm. Therefore, each microbeam ablates a volume of 0.05 $mm^3$ of scarred tissue, and calculating this ablation for thousands of times, a great amount of scarred tissue can be removed. At the same time, the thin columns break the disorganized thick collagen fibrils that create the contracture. The mechanical forces that create the contracture are immediately

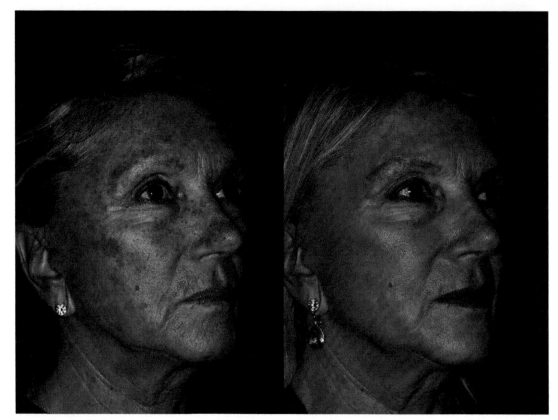

**Fig. 9.** Result of a fractional resurfacing of the face using the multilayer technique (8-month follow-up).

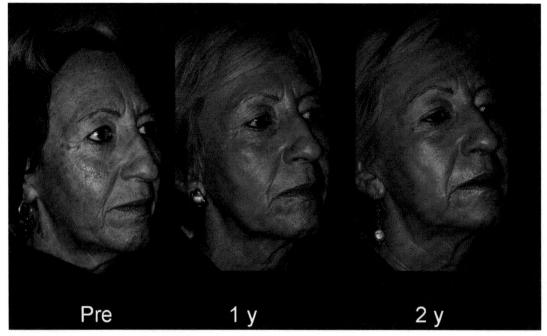

Pre                    1 y                    2 y

**Fig. 10.** Result of a fractional resurfacing of the face (2-year follow-up).

interrupted, and the body has the ability to heal in a more organized fashion. We are convinced that the ablation of the scar tissue as well as the interruption of the contraction forces are the explanation why patients refer, immediately after the procedure, a relaxation of the scars the patients refer immediately after the procedure. The ablation of the scar tissue and the interruption of the contraction forces are not the only aspect involved in the final relaxation of a scar. The result thus obtained could be frustrated by a subsequent further healing process. Interacting with the skin, the laser energy also determines heat release. A controlled (this is why a very short-pulse duration $CO_2$ laser is preferable to longer-pulse duration devices) heat diffusion induces a molecular cascade, including heat-shock proteins and matrix metalloproteinases (MMP) as well as inflammatory processes that lead to a rapid healing response and prolonged neocollagenesis with subsequent collagen remodeling. Studies on the effect of fractional $CO_2$ laser on scar have shown alterations of types I and III procollagen; MMP-1; transforming growth factor-b2, -b3, and -bFGF, and miRNAs miR-18a and miR-19a expressions.[7] In a subsequent study, gene expression profiling revealed induced expression of Wnt5a, CYR61, and HSP90 in human skin during the early remodeling phase after fractional $CO_2$ laser treatment.[8] All these proteins play an important role in collagen remodeling. It was demonstrated that after an ultrapulse fractional $CO_2$ procedure, there is an inversion of the ratio between collagen type I and collagen type III. Although some MMPs' production is upregulated, profibrotic growth factors are downregulated. Ultrapulse fractional $CO_2$ procedures also produce a dermal architecture change. Collagen fibers are less thick, and the classical organization parallel to the surface is much less evident. Collagen fibers are more chaotic (more similar to normal skin), and also the vascularity is different. After the procedure, there are more vessels of small calibers oriented vertically.[9]

## PREOPERATIVE EVALUATION AND SETUP

All scarring areas should be carefully observed, and patients should be forced to perform movements pointing out eventual retractive bands. A careful marking of the entire region that will be treated with a skin marker will allow for the procedure to be performed faster. Retractive bands as well as atrophic areas must be marked. The authors do not prescribe any prophylactic drugs if small areas will be treated, whereas huge areas require, in the authors' opinion, an antiviral, an antibiotic, and an antifungal prophylactic therapy.

The drugs are the same of those described before. Procedures on small areas (up to 500 $cm^2$) can be performed by applying a topical anesthetic cream (the authors use Pliaglis, Galderma, which is composed by lidocaine 7% and tetracaine 7%) and using a cold air chiller device (Cryo 6; Zimmer) to attempt to reduce the discomfort of the patients during the procedure. An ultrasound evaluation of the scar establishing the thickness in the different areas of it can be very helpful in deciding on the energy that could be applied on different areas.

## THE PROCEDURE

All scars can clinically present thick areas, atrophic areas, and many superficial irregularities. All these aspects must be addressed during each single procedure. There also are no standardized settings because scars are extremely different regarding thickness, pliability, and superficial features. A few general rules should be always, in the authors opinion, followed:

- Ablated microcolumns must penetrate the full thickness of the scar without getting to the subcutaneous tissue.
- The higher the energy applied, the lower the density of the microcolumns.
- Oppositely, the lower the energy applied, the higher the density of the microcolumns.
- Pinpoint bleeding can be considered a good clinical end point.
- A visible contraction of the scar tissue during the procedures should be carefully avoided.

Our protocol can be divided into three distinct steps for simplicity.

The authors start the laser session (step 1; **Fig. 11**) by treating the thicker areas/bands using the microablation hand piece. It creates microcolumns with a diameter of 120 $\mu$m and of variable penetration according to the energy. An energy of 150 mJ creates a penetration of around 4.0 mm, whereas an energy of 100 mJ creates a penetration of 2.6 mm.

The proper energy level to apply is the one that is able to create ablated columns of depth slightly below the thickness of the scar. Using magnification lenses, the authors observe the interaction of the laser with the scar during the first couple of shots. If a contraction of the tissue is observed, the energy level will be reduced. The correct threshold of energy to apply is the one that, impacting the skin, creates a column of ablation without any contraction (or creates a minimal contraction). Pinpoint bleeding is also a second good end point to achieve. Very thick scars are usually treated with an energy of 150 mJ and a

# Step 1

**Microablation handpiece**
**Energy up to 150 mJ**
**Density 1% – 3% for collagen remodeling**
**Density 10% – 20 % for collagen production**

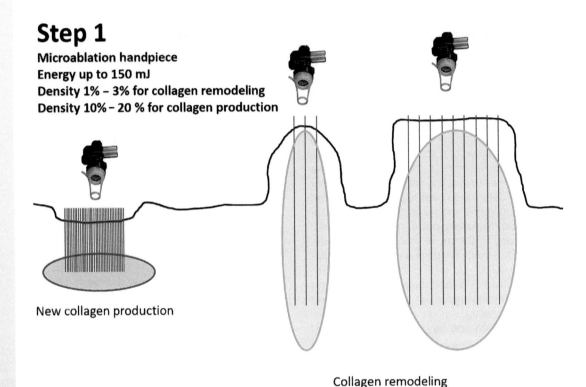

New collagen production

Collagen remodeling

**Fig. 11.** Step 1 of the treatment of atrophic (*left*) and thick scars (*right*).

density of 1%, whereas atrophic areas can be treated with an energy of 30 to 35 mJ and a density of 5% to 10%. The authors suggestion is to always change the energy level according to the skin reaction.

The deep previous procedure is followed by a much more superficial one (step 2; **Fig. 12**). The authors use the CPG hand piece, applying very low energy (30–50 mJ), very high frequency (350–400 Hz), very high density of microbeams (very high density with an overlap of more than 50%), and a very small hexagonal spot.

With these settings, the authors sculpt all superficial irregularities they can observe. The correct end point is to observe a white ablation of the surface. Brown and dark-brown color must not be

# Step 2

**CPG handpiece – very small spot size**
**Energy 30 – 50 mJ**
**Density up to 9 (more than 50% overlapping)**
**Frequency  350 Hz – 400 Hz**

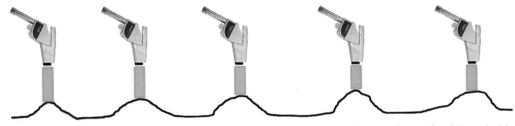

**Fig. 12.** Step 2 of the procedure. Using low energy and high frequency and density, all superficial irregularities are treated.

# Step 3

**CPG handpiece – biggest spot size**
**Energy 125 mJ – 150 mJ**
**Density up to 3 (max 82% of coverage)**
**Frequency  125 Hz – 150 Hz**

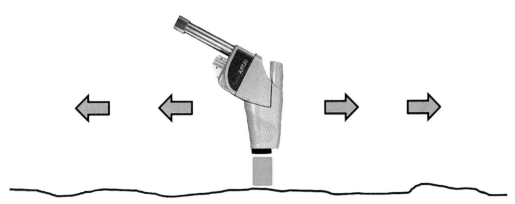

**Fig. 13.** Step 3 of the procedure. A conventional fractional procedure is performed on the full scarred area.

observed (brown and dark brown means deeper penetration and more release of heat), and if this happens, the energy must be reduced.

At the end of the procedure, the authors cover the full extent of the scarred area (step 3; **Fig. 13**) using the same hand piece used in step 2 but modifying the settings. They increase to the maximum the dimension of the shot, reduce the energy to 125 to 150 mJ, reduce the density using coverage of around 80%, and reduce the frequency to 125 to 150 Hz. This pure fractional pass has the aim of obtaining a better and uniform superficial appearance.

Since 2009, we started to treat patients with mature scars (older than 2 years without evidence of evolution). However, our practice has now changed to treating patients as soon as possible after the acute burn phase. Our combined experience strongly suggests that the fractional $CO_2$ laser promotes a normalisation of the healing process, when laser is applied close to naturally remodelling wounds. Conseqently our practice has change to treating patients as soon as possible after the acute burn phase.[10–12]

The authors cannot say how many sessions are required to obtain a very good result (**Figs. 14** and **15**), but are convinced that a good outcome can be achieved just after the first session, but also that more sessions can obtain a better result. The authors clinical results confirmed what was already published,[7,13–33] allowing them to affirm that lasers may disrupt old algorithms on scar treatments and reset their expectations of what can be achieved, in terms of restoring form and

function in burn patients. Fractional $CO_2$ treatment induces also strong improvements in the patient's quality of life, and although it does not replace reconstructive surgery, it may well decrease the extent of subsequent surgical procedures and prepares the scar for an optimal outcome.

## POSTOPERATIVE MANAGEMENT

Immediately after the laser procedure, the entire treated area is covered with wet cold sterile gauzes. A nurse applies drops of cold saline solution on the gauzes every 3 to 5 minutes to keep them wet. The same nurse continues to use the cold air chilling device on the full treated area for 5 to 10 minutes after the procedure. When the pain and the burning feeling disappears (10–20 minutes after the procedure), the wet gauzes are removed and a silicone gel (Stratamed; Stratpharma, Basel, Switzerland) is applied on the full area. The patient is instructed to apply a thin layer of the same cream at least 2 times per day for the next 4 to 7 days (or until all crusts disappear) and to have a shower the evening of the day after the procedure (a gentle cleanser is allowed). Finally, the patient is instructed not to expose the treated area to UV rays and to apply an SPF 50+ at least every 4 hours when outside for the 2 months after the procedure.

## ADVERSE EVENTS

The authors believe that proper preparation as well as optimal postoperative procedures can reduce the incidence of adverse events. Major adverse

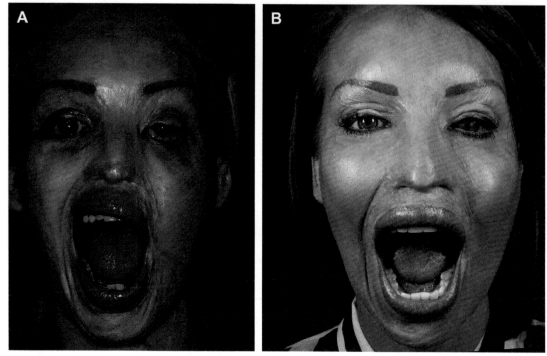

**Fig. 14.** A severe acid burn (*A*) before and (*B*) after 3 sessions of treatment.

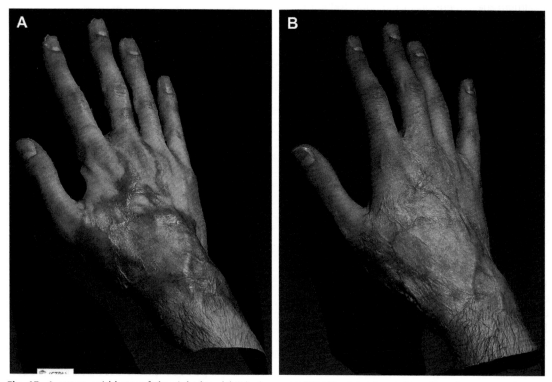

**Fig. 15.** A severe acid burn of the right hand (*A*) before and (*B*) after 3 sessions of treatment.

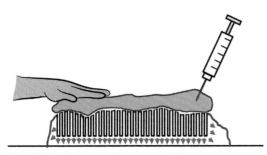

**Fig. 16.** The laser-assisted drug delivery.

events, like new scars formation, have never been observed, and these data confirmed what was previously published.[9] The authors do not consider erythema, oozing, and swelling for the first 2 days adverse events. They should be considered a normal evolution of the healing process. The authors incidence of hypopigmentation and hyperpigmentation is extremely low in contrast with what already published,[34] but they believe that this low incidence does not depend on technique but on the fair-skinned patients' population.

### The Laser-Assisted Drug Delivery

Burn scars management with laser is expanding very quickly, but 1 aspect is developing faster. The fractional Co$_2$ can be used as a drug delivery system. Fractional laser therapy creates precise, uniform columns of tissue vaporization, which facilitate drug delivery past the epidermal barrier and evenly distribute drugs in the dermal layer. The technique is very simple and consists of performing the already described procedure on scars, immediately followed by the application of a mix of drugs just on the top of the treated areas **(Fig. 16)**.

This fluid cocktail has only to be massaged on the scar until its complete absorption. This concept has been shown in several animal models to enhance the bioavailability of topically applied drugs,[35–37] and the use of laser-assisted delivery of corticosteroid in scars has been reported in some case series.[38,39] The authors usually prepare a cocktail of drugs containing 5-fluorouracil (5FU), triamcinolone (TAC), and Botulinum toxin, and they changed the percentage of each of them accordingly with the scar features. In trying to simplify the concept, they use a high percentages of 5FU for the thickness, high percentages of TAC for the inflammation (and the authors always use a mix of these 2 drugs), and they add botulinum toxin if a fast proliferation rate of the scar is appreciated.[40,41]

## REFERENCES

1. Walsh JT Jr, Thomas J, Flotte TJ, et al. Pulsed CO2 laser tissue ablation: effect of tissue type and pulse duration on thermal damage. Lasers Surg Med 1988;8(2):108–18.
2. Ross VE, Domankevitz Y, Skrobal M, et al. Effects of CO2 laser pulse duration in ablation and residual thermal damage: implications for skin resurfacing. Lasers Surg Med 1996;19(2):123–9.
3. Farkas JP, Richardson JA, Brown SA, et al. TUNEL assay to characterize acute histopathological injury following treatment with the active and deep FX fractional short-pulse CO2 devices. Aesthet Surg J 2010;30(4):603–13.
4. Dover JS, Bhatia AC, Stewart B, et al. Topical 5-aminolevulinic acid combined with intense pulsed light in the treatment of photoaging. Arch Dermatol 2005;141:1247–52.
5. Clementoni MT, Gilardino P, Muti GF, et al. Non-sequential fractional ultrapulsed CO2 resurfacing of photoaged facial skin: preliminary clinical report. J Cosmet Laser Ther 2007;9(4):218–25.
6. Tretti Clementoni M, Galimberti M, Tourlaki A, et al. Random fractional ultrapulsed CO2 resurfacing of photodamaged facial skin: long-term evaluation. Lasers Med Sci 2013;28(2):643–50.
7. Qu L, Liu A, Zhou L, et al. Clinical and molecular effects on mature burn scars after treatment with a fractional CO2 laser. Lasers Surg Med 2012;44:517–24.
8. Hu Y, Chen Y, Lin M, et al. Pathogenic role of the Wnt signaling pathway activation in laser-induced choroidal neovascularization. Invest Ophthalmol Vis Sci 2013;54:141–54.
9. Connolly KL, Chaffins M, Ozog D. Vascular patterns in mature hypertrophic burn scars treated with fractional CO2 laser. Lasers Surg Med 2014;46(8):597–600.
10. Karmisholt KE, Banzhaf CA, Glud M, et al. Laser treatments in early wound healing improve scar appearance: a randomized split-wound trial with nonablative fractional laser exposures vs. untreated controls. Br J Dermatol 2018;179(6):1307–14.
11. Karmisholt KE, Haerskjold A, Karlsmark T, et al. Early laser intervention to reduce scar formation–a systematic review. J Eur Acad Dermatol Venereol 2018;32(7):1099–110.
12. Yang Z, Lv Y, Yue F, et al. Early intervention of fractional carbon dioxide laser on fresh traumatic scar. Lasers Med Sci 2019;34(7):1317–24.
13. Hultman CS, Friedstat JS, Edkins RE, et al. Laser resurfacing and remodeling of hypertrophic burn scars: the results of a large, prospective, before-after cohort study, with long-term follow-up. Ann Surg 2014;260(3):519–29 [discussion: 529–32].
14. Cervelli V, Gentile P, Spallone D, et al. Ultrapulsed fractional CO2 laser for the treatment of post-traumatic and pathological scars. J Drugs Dermatol 2010;9(11):1328–31.

15. Uebelhoer NS, Ross EV, Shumaker PR. Ablative fractional resurfacing for the treatment of traumatic scars and contractures. Semin Cutan Med Surg 2012;31(2).110–20.

16. Waibel J, Beer K. Ablative fractional laser resurfacing for the treatment of a third-degree burn. J Drugs Dermatol 2009;8(3):294–7.

17. Hultman CS, Edkins RE, Lee CN, et al. Shine on: review of laser- and light-based therapies for the treatment of burn scars. Dermatol Res Pract 2012;2012: 243651.

18. Gold MH, Berman B, Clementoni MT, et al. International advisory panel on scar management. Updated international clinical recommendations on scar management: part 1—evaluating the evidence. Dermatol Surg 2014;40:817–24.

19. Gold MH, McGuire M, Mustoe TA, et al. International advisory panel on scar management updated international clinical recommendations on scar management: part 2—algorithms for scar prevention and treatment. Dermatol Surg 2014;40:825–31.

20. Anzarut A, Olson J, Singh P, et al. The effectiveness of pressure garment therapy for the prevention of abnormal scarring after burn injury: a meta-analysis. J Plast Reconstr Aesthet Surg 2009;62:77–84.

21. Levi B, Ibrahim A, Mathews K, et al. The use of CO2 fractional photothermolysis for the treatment of burn scars. J Burn Care Res 2016;37(2):106–14.

22. Issler-Fisher AC, Fisher OM, Smialkowski AO, et al. Ablative fractional CO2 laser for burn scar reconstruction: an extensive subjective and objective short-term outcome analysis of a prospective treatment cohort. Burns 2017;43(3):573–82.

23. Anderson RR, Donelan MB, Hivnor C, et al. Laser treatment of traumatic scars with an emphasis on ablative fractional laser resurfacing: consensus report. JAMA Dermatol 2014;150(2):187–93.

24. Waibel J, Beer K. Fractional laser resurfacing for thermal burns. J Drugs Dermatol 2008;7:59–61.

25. Willows BM, Ilyas M, Sharma A. Laser in the management of burn scars. Burns 2017. https://doi.org/10.1016/j.burns.2017.07.001 [pii:S0305-4179(17)30376-5].

26. El-Zawahry BM, Sobhi RM, Bassiouny DA, et al. Ablative CO2 fractional resurfacing in treatment of thermal burn scars: an open-label controlled clinical and histopathological study. J Cosmet Dermatol 2015;14(4):324–31.

27. Khandelwal A, Yelvington M, Tang X, et al. Ablative fractional photothermolysis for the treatment of hypertrophic burn scars in adult and pediatric patients: a single surgeon's experience. J Burn Care Res 2014;35:455–63.

28. Haedersdal M. Fractional ablative CO2 laser resurfacing improves a thermal burn scar. J Eur Acad Dermatol Venereol 2009;23:1327–49.

29. Lee SJ, Kim JH, Lee SE, et al. Hypertrophic scarring after burn scar treatment with a 10,600-nm carbon dioxide fractional laser. Dermatol Surg 2011;37: 1168–72.

30. Krakowski AC, Admani S, Shumaker PR, et al. Fractionated carbon dioxide laser as a novel, noninvasive treatment approach to burn scar-related nail dystrophy. Dermatol Surg 2014;40(3):351–4.

31. Shumaker PR, Kwan JM, Landers JT, et al. Functional improvements in traumatic scars and scar contractures using an ablative fractional laser protocol. J Trauma Acute Care Surg 2012;73:S116–21.

32. Krakowski AC, Goldenber A, Eichenfield LF, et al. Ablative fractional laser resurfacing helps treat restrictive pediatric scar contractures. Pediatrics 2014;134:1700–5.

33. Poetschke J, Dornseifer U, Clementoni MT, et al. Ultrapulsed fractional ablative carbon dioxide laser treatment of hypertrophic burn scars: evaluation of an in-patient controlled, standardized treatment approach. Lasers Med Sci 2017;32(5): 1031–40.

34. Clayton JL, Edkins R, Cairns BA, et al. Incidence and management of adverse events after the use of laser therapies for the treatment of hypertrophic burn scars. Ann Plast Surg 2013;70:500–5.

35. Haedersdal M, Sakamoto FH, Farinelli WA, et al. Fractional CO(2) laser-assisted drug delivery. Lasers Surg Med 2010;42(2):113–22.

36. Forster B, Klein A, Szeimies RM, et al. Penetration enhancement of two topical 5-aminolaevulinic acid formulations for photodynamic therapy by erbium: YAG laser ablation of the stratum corneum: continuous versus fractional ablation. Exp Dermatol 2010;19(9):806–12.

37. Lee WR, Shen SC, Pai MH, et al. Fractional laser as a tool to enhance the skin permeation of 5-aminolevulinic acid with minimal skin disruption: a comparison with conventional erbium:YAG laser. J Control Release 2010;145(2):124–33.

38. Waibel JS, Wulkan AJ, Shumaker PR. Treatment of hypertrophic scars using laser and laser assisted corticosteroid delivery. Lasers Surg Med 2013; 45(3):135–40.

39. Cavalie MSL, Montaudie H, Bahadoran P, et al. Treatment of keloids with laser-assisted topical steroid delivery: a retrospective study of 23 cases. Dermatol Ther 2015;28:74–8.

40. Austin E, Koo E, Jagdeo J. The cellular response of keloids and hypertrophic scars to botulinum toxin A: a comprehensive literature review. Dermatol Surg 2018;44(2):149–57.

41. Chen HC, Yen CI, Yang SY, et al. Comparison of steroid and botulinum toxin type A monotherapy with combination therapy for treating human hypertrophic scars in an animal model. Plast Reconstr Surg 2017;140(1):43e–9e.

# Broad Band Light and Skin Rejuvenation

Patrick Bitter Jr, MD, FAAD

## KEYWORDS

- Broad band light • Skin rejuvenation • Pulsed light

## KEY POINTS

- Over the past 25 years, broad spectrum pulsed light has established its place in aesthetics and laser medicine.
- Pulsed light has proven its usefulness, effectiveness, and versatility in treating a multitude of skin problems, delaying skin aging, maintaining healthy skin, and as an adjunct to a cosmetic surgical practice for noninvasive skin rejuvenation and in the treatment of postsurgical scars.
- Practitioners contemplating adding a pulsed light device to their practice should choose a device that has at least 4 important features: (1) a large spot size, (2) variable-sized smaller spot adaptors, (3) pulse rates of at least 1 pulse per second, (4) a wide range of cutoff filters, including 515 nm, 560 nm, 590 nm, 640 nm, and 695 nm to treat most skin types.

## INTRODUCTION AND EARLY HISTORY OF INTENSE PULSED LIGHT

Pulsed light energy devices for medical and aesthetic use were initially developed in the early 1990s. Pulsed light referred as intense pulsed light, or IPL, was the product of the Israeli medical device manufacturer, Israeli Company Energy Systems Corporation (ESC [Yokneam, Israel]).

The first broad spectrum pulsed light device was introduced in the early 1990s by ESC. The first IPL was branded PhotoDerm. This initial IPL device used a xenon flash lamp that emitted a pulse of light in the visible and infrared spectrum. This light would be filtered using specially coated cutoff filters. The early filters worked by blocking shorter wavelengths of light so the skin was exposed to wavelengths of light above the cutoff filter. Cutoff filters of 515 nm, 560 nm, and 590 nm were available to the practitioner.

In addition, the practitioner could vary the pulse duration and interpulse interval, delivering a train of up to 3 consecutive pulses. The practitioner could adjust the energy fluence with maximum fluences up to 45 J on the PhotoDerm.

The initial device did not offer contact cooling. The initial IPL device had a single spot size and repetition rate of 9 seconds. This initial IPL design: xenon flash lamps, cutoff filters, high maximum fluences, and ability to vary the pulse durations, has formed the basis of the designs of the successor IPL technologies. A specific IPL from ESC was Food and Drug Administration approved for the specific treatment of leg telangiectasis.

The initial experience with IPL in the United States was mixed, with many practitioners finding the results of leg vein treatments to be unsuccessful and often problematic, causing superficial burns and hypopigmented and hyperpigmented crystal coloration in the rectangular shape of the treatment.

Indeed, by 1998, the US experience with IPL, although limited to less than 200 practices across the country, was mainly a negative view of IPL for its approved indication of the treatment of leg veins.

Some laser experts maintained that IPL had no place in dermatology or laser medicine or aesthetics. Indeed, ESC was facing a class action lawsuit filed by a group of physicians alleging the

Dermatology, Advanced Aesthetic Dermatology, 16400 Lark Avenue, Suite 300, Los Gatos, CA 95032, USA
*E-mail address:* bitterjrmd@aol.com

Facial Plast Surg Clin N Am 28 (2020) 29–36
https://doi.org/10.1016/j.fsc.2019.09.014
1064-7406/20/© 2019 Elsevier Inc. All rights reserved.

technology was not represented accurately as an effective treatment for leg veins.

At the same time, some IPL practitioners were individually recognizing that IPL could result in hair reduction and was also effective for some benign pigmented skin lesions, such as lentigines and freckles and small facial vessels.

## EARLY OBSERVATIONS

These early observations were based on the spot treatment approach, whereby only 1 area of the face with visible vessels or pigmented spots or areas of undesired hair growth were treated. These early treatments typically were a single pulse over the affected area. During this same time period, it began to be appreciated that IPL was most suited for fairer skin types (Fitzpatrick skin types I through III). It was also observed that complications of superficial burns resulting in hypopigmentation and hyperpigmentation were most common when tanned skin or darker skin types were treated.

Some IPL practitioners maintained that IPL was not a suitable technology for ethnic skin types or any skin type beyond Fitzpatrick skin type III. Other IPL practitioners found that by reducing the fluence, using higher-numbered cutoff filters, and lengthening the pulse durations, some patients with skin types IV and V could have pigmented spots treated or hair removed. Problems still occurred, however, because the initial crystal size was often much larger than the size of the target vessel or pigmented spot even when the settings were more conservative. The result left an area the shape of the crystal spot size that contrasted with the surrounding untreated skin.

During this time, there was a growing awareness among IPL practitioners that IPL was useful in the right patient population for fair-skinned individuals, for hair removal, and for select and benign pigmented and vascular lesions, primarily of the face. It was not until the initial presentation and introduction in August 1998 at an International Dermatology Conference in Athens, Greece by the author, describing a technique of using IPL as a full facial treatment and performing a series of sequential treatments, that IPL truly gained traction as a potentially useful treatment for photoaged skin. The author's results of this technique as a series of full-face IPL treatments for photorejuvenation was published in *Dermatologic Surgery*.[1]

The results of this treatment presented by the author demonstrated the gradual clearing of many of the signs of photo damage: freckling, fine wrinkles, larger pores, as well as erythema and telangiectasis, without the downtime that was seen with the ablative carbon dioxide and Erbium:YAG lasers. Even the widely used pulse dye laser for vascular lesions produced purpura at treatment sites that could take up to 10 days or more to resolve.

Over the next 20 years, IPL has evolved to become a well-accepted multimodality technology for skin rejuvenation and treatment of vascular and pigmented lesions and for hair removal.

There are now more than 2 dozen companies worldwide that manufacture IPL devices. The original company, ESC, has evolved to become Lumenis. There are estimated to be well over ten thousand IPL devices worldwide, and more than ten thousand IPL practitioners at the time of this publication. It is probable that more than 20,000 IPL treatments are performed daily in the United States alone.

## PRESENT DAY ACCEPTED USES OF PULSED LIGHT ENERGY DEVICES

There have been several key innovations in pulsed light technology and techniques that have been introduced during the past 20 years that have resulted in improved treatment results, reduced complications, faster treatment times, and new clinical applications. In the author's opinion, the most important innovations in technology have been (1) faster repetition rates, (2) larger spot sizes, (3) variable-sized spot adaptors to allow a focused spot treatment of small vascular and pigmented lesions, (4) contact cooling, (5) a continual pulsed mode, and (6) expanded spectrum of cutoff filters.

Faster repetition rates have made for more practical treatment of large skin areas. Areas, such as arms, legs, back, and treatments of face, neck, and chest can now be treated at a single session in a fraction of the time it took to treat with the original IPL device. Repetition rates of up to 3 Hz are now available. Larger spot size combined with these faster repetition rates has reduced treatment times for large areas from an hour or more to 10 minutes or less.

Variable-sized spot adapters that were the innovation of Sciton Medical (Palo Alto, CA, USA), affixed to the large spot crystal, have allowed the focused targeting of small vessels and small pigmented lesions with much higher and more effective settings that could otherwise cause a complication if the large spot size was used. In addition, spot adaptors as small as 3 mm have made possible the treatment of lesions in locations such as the canthus, lower lids, alar folds, and ears.

The innovation of constant cooling of the crystal to temperatures as low as 0°C (Sciton Medical; BBL) as a means to protect the epidermis when higher fluences are used has reduced the complications of superficial burns while making treatments more comfortable for patients.

The availability of up to 7 different filters (Sciton Medical), including 420, 515, 560, 590, 640, 695, and 800, to the practitioner has expanded the range of skin types to now include the treatment of even skin type 6 (the darkest skin type on the Fitzpatrick scale) possible. The cutoff filter functions to change the spectrum. By choosing the appropriate cutoff filter, which alters the light spectrum of the xenon flash lamp, the proper fluence, pulse duration, and contact cooling, all skin types can now be safely treated.

Finally, the continual pulse mode innovation introduced by Sciton in 2008 for the purpose of skin tightening has become an exciting technology not just for nonsurgical skin tightening, but also for a growing spectrum of new clinical applications of broad spectrum light that were previously not possible.

## KEY INNOVATIONS IN TREATMENT, RESEARCH, AND EDUCATION

The key technique innovations of pulsed light technology are as follows:

1. A multiple-pass technique (as developed by the author)
2. A 2-step technique for skin correction and photo-rejuvenation (as developed by the author)
3. Observing and recording the pulse counts for each treatment. The recording of pulse counts for each step of the treatment has led to more consistent predictable and reproducible outcomes, fewer complications, better results, and reduced learning curves.
4. Performing enough treatments (as developed by the author). Initial efforts with IPL were focused on the goals of eliminating vascular or pigmented lesions in a single treatment session.

With time and experience, it became clear that attempting to clear vascular and pigmented lesions in a single treatment session was often not realistic and that more than 1 treatment was necessary.

By taking the multiple-pass treatment approach, expected outcomes were more realistically achieved. Setting a patient's expectations at 3 to 5 treatment sessions in practice was more realistic and allowed for the first treatment session to be more conservative, reducing the 2 most common IPL complications, superficial burns and lack of results.

Another benefit that has come from multiple treatments is the observation that results, in particular, for clarity and textural improvements, were progressive and that the people with the clearest, smoothest, healthiest-appearing skin were those who typically had the most treatments.

Several factors have contributed to the widespread popularity and common use of IPL and broad spectrum light devices. First was the introduction of a technique using IPL for overall skin rejuvenation that was based on a series of full-face or a series of nonfacial skin treatments.

The concept that IPL was well suited as a technology for noninvasive overall rejuvenation of photo-aged skin using a technique of serial, sequential, full-face (or nonfacial) skin treatments was first reported by the author.[1] This landmark study reported on the observations for 49 subjects of the effective rejuvenation of photo-damaged skin using a series of full-face IPL treatments.

One of the major observations reported by the author was that the photo-damaged skin, pigmented lesions, erythema, telangiectasis, and fine wrinkles could be effectively improved with essentially no downtime and minimal complications. Histology of treated skin showed reduced superficial vasculature, reduced dermal melanin, increased collagen, and reduced dermal inflammation. This breakthrough treatment was a major impetus for medical device manufacturers to develop and market pulsed light devices.

Second, with more energy-based device manufacturers introducing pulsed light devices with more advanced features, such as more rapid pulse rates, larger spot sizes, preprogrammed parameters as well as contact cooling, at increasingly more affordable prices, the availability of IPL treatments became more widespread.

Third, educational efforts undertaken largely by the author and Dr Steven Mulholland in treatment techniques, parameters, and various applications of IPL trained several thousand early IPL adaptors and users from 2000 to 2010. These early educational events taught effective IPL techniques and marketing strategies to not only physicians in the core aesthetic specialties of plastic and facial plastics, dermatology, and ophthalmology, but also to many noncore physicians who were making their first foray into a cash-based aesthetic medicine practice.

In addition, many US states allowed nonphysicians to operate IPL devices. Early IPL training events also included many nurses, aestheticians, and nonmedical laser technicians. Another benefit of these early IPL educational events was to dispel the misconceptions and myths of IPL that had deterred the early adoption of IPL as having a legitimate place in laser medicine.

Finally, because of the generally favorable and patient-pleasing outcomes of IPL treatments, the popularity of IPL treatments grew substantially. In 2019, more than 30 laser device manufacturers now offer an IPL device.

## PRESENT USES OF INTENSE PULSED LIGHT TECHNOLOGY IN AESTHETIC AND LASER MEDICINE

The present well-accepted and common uses of pulsed light include both corrective and adjunctive benefits. The author has developed advanced courses on both IPL and broad spectrum light treatment methodology that he continues to teach today to educated users on treatment methodology, including Corrective Benefits of Pulsed Light Technology, Adjunctive Benefits of Pulsed Light Technology, and Future Uses of Pulsed Light Technology.

Corrective Benefits of Pulsed Light Technology include the following: (1) noninvasive photo-rejuvenation of photo-damaged facial and nonfacial skin; (2) treatment of vascular and erythematous conditions, including rosacea, poikiloderma, general erythema, telangiectasis, and benign pigmented lesions; (3) acne; (4) scars and purpura; (5) hair reduction and removal; (6) delay of skin aging; (7) wrinkle reduction; and (8) skin-laxity and skin-tightening treatment.

The adjunctive benefits of Pulsed Light Technology include the following: (1) the early treatment of post surgical scarring and red, raised surgical scars, (2) ecchymosis and purpura post-procedure, (3) postlaser erythema, and (4) post-inflammatory hyperpigmentation.

Of the well accepted clinical and aesthetic benefits of pulsed light treatments, rejuvenation of photo-damaged skin and improvement in the symptoms of rosacea are the 2 most common applications of pulsed light.

## PHOTO-REJUVENATION WITH PULSED LIGHT

Since the introduction of the serial full-face technique with IPL in 2000 by the author, photo-rejuvenation of photo-damaged skin has become the most popular and widely accepted use of pulsed light. Most of the signs of chronic sun exposure, such as freckling, fine wrinkling, telangiectasis, erythema, and larger pores, are visibly improved with a series of pulsed light treatments.

The recommended technique for consistent, predictable, and reproducible results is a multiple-pass, 2-step technique. With this technique, the first step is performed as 2 passes using conservative parameters. Typically, a 515-nm or 560-nm cutoff filter is used for Fitzpatrick skin types I through III, and 590 nm for Fitzpatrick skin types IV. Lower fluence, generally less than 10 J cm, depending on the specific device, is used.

The purpose of the first step is to produce a general overall clearing of freckled pigmentation and a smoother texture to the skin. The first step is responsible for stimulating new dermal collagen, producing favorable gene expression changes in keratinocytes and dermal fibroblasts. It is the first step that results in clearer, smoother, healthier-appearing skin as well as providing antiaging benefits.

By performing 2 passes at lower fluences, the complications of uneven striping and superficial burns are largely eliminated.

The second step of this technique uses higher fluences and smaller spot sizes to specifically target telangiectasis, areas of erythema, stubborn pigmented lesions, wrinkles, and scars that may not resolve as effectively with the lower fluences used in step 1.

The advantages of the multiple-pass, 2-step technique for photo-rejuvenation over the early single-pass, high-fluence technique are better overall results, greater textural improvements, and elimination of complications, such as uneven results, striping, superficial burns, and lack of results. In addition, the multiple-pass, 2-step technique is more comfortable for patients. Depending on the device used, typical full-face treatments with this technique may be 240 to 400 pulses.

This same technique is used to treat any nonfacial photo-aged skin. The most popular are the neck, chest, and dorsal hands.

## TREATMENT OF ROSACEA, ERYTHEMA, TELANGIECTASIAS

Although the early experience with IPL for spider leg veins was not successful, the treatment of rosacea with its various symptoms of telangiectasia and erythema is highly successful with pulsed light. Indeed, the author's experience with IPL and broad spectrum light in several thousand patients for rosacea has shown high success rates of up to 90% to 100% resolution of erythema and flushing for periods of up to 5 or more years following a series of 5 treatments.

The author uses the multiple-pass, 2-step technique (as developed by the author) for facial rosacea and erythema of the neck (Poikiloderma

Civatte) and décolleté. The author has observed that all symptoms of rosacea, including erythema, flushing, burning, telangiectasis, inflammatory papules, and ocular rosacea, improve with a series of full-face pulsed light treatments. Typical parameters for step 2 for rosacea use the 560-nm filter for Fitzpatrick skin types I through III and 590-nm filter for skin types IV. Higher fluences, such as 15 to 18 J, with the Sciton BroadBand Light (BBL) device are used. It is recommended to use an additional external cooling for this step to help increase patient comfort and reduce posttreatment swelling.

Although rosacea symptoms improve dramatically with pulsed light treatments, the author recommends a maintenance treatment every 6 months to keep patients symptom free. Also, 25% of rosacea patients may need more than 5 treatments to achieve 75% or greater reduction in erythema and flushing.

In 2019, pulsed light treatments continue to be one of the most effective and valuable treatments for rosacea, general erythema, and flushing.

## TREATMENT OF ACNE WITH PULSED LIGHT

Another inflammatory condition that has proven to respond well to pulsed light treatments is acne vulgaris.

The author published a paper describing a 3-step technique using BBL to simultaneously treat both inflammatory acne and acne vulgaris.[2]

The first step is 5 to 6 passes using the blue spectrum of light (420 nm to 480 nm). This narrow band of blue light spectrum is achieved using a specially coated filter. The purpose of the blue light step is the reduction of new inflammatory acne lesions.

The second step is 2 passes using the 560-nm cutoff filter (590-nm cutoff filter for Fitzpatrick skin types IV) and similar parameters that are used for the treatment of rosacea (560 nm, 15 J cm, 15 milliseconds, 15° contact cooling with the broad spectrum light device). The purpose of this step is the simultaneous resolution of active acne and improvements in erythematous and violaceous raised or depressed scars.

A third step using an innovative continual pulsed mode setting (Skintyte, BBL device; Sciton) results in rapid resolution of active acne and reduction of new acne lesions. Results with this multiple-pass 3-step technique are very rapid resolution of active inflammatory papules and cysts (1 to 7 days) and reduction in erythematous acne scars. Indeed, if the acne scar is erythematous and elevated or depressed, it becomes smoother and less erythematous.

Results in a series of 100 patients have shown complete to nearly complete resolution of inflammatory acne, including cystic acne in 80% of patients with a series of 8 weekly or biweekly treatments. Remission of inflammatory acne can be up to 6 months after the last treatment. The 3 primary benefits of pulsed light for acne using this 3-step technique are as follows: (1) rapid resolution of inflammatory acne, (2) improvement in erythematous scars, and (3) a nondrug treatment option for people with inflammatory acne. Although relapse of inflammatory acne may occur after 3 months, improvement in acne scarring is permanent.

## TREATMENT OF SCARRING WITH PULSED LIGHT

Pulsed light is very effective in improving the erythematous, violaceous, or hyperpigmented scars. In the author's experience, the sooner a newly formed scar is treated, the better the aesthetic improvement. Pulsed light is especially effective in the early treatment of new surgical scars. The author recommends initiating the first pulsed light treatment on a facial surgical scar at 1 week after suture removal and 2 weeks after suture removal for nonfacial scars. When a scar is in the erythematous stage, pulsed light treatments are especially efficacious to reduce the erythema and flatten an elevated scar or fill in a depressed scar.

It is the author's practice to treat all surgical scars with pulsed light at the earliest time. It is the author's contention that pulsed light should be regarded as the first line of treatment of choice for surgical scars. Early intervention with pulsed light may help prevent a hypertrophic or keloid scar.

The technique used for treating surgical or traumatic scars is 2 to 3 passes over the scar overlapping pulses 10% to 20%. The most effective parameters for scars are those used to treat erythema and telangiectasis for rosacea. The smaller spot sizes that are approximately the width or size of a scar are chosen over the largest spot size unless a scar is particularly large. The author recommends a series of 3 to 4 pulsed light treatments with 1 treatment every 3 to 4 weeks.

Scars that have been successfully treated are facial and body excisional scars, hypertrophic scars, breast surgery scars, abdominoplasty scars, brachioplasty scars, full- and split-thickness skin grafts, liposuction scars, burn scars, radiation scars, orthopedic scars, and hypertrophic scars over joints (elbows, ankles, knees, fingers). In general, the response to pulsed light of all these various scars is similar with gradual fading of erythema and smoothing of the scar over several weeks. Pulsed light is effective on new scars and avoids further injury to a healing wound as occurs with ablative and fractionated scars and microneedling devices. It should be an essential tool in an aesthetic surgeon's practice.

## HAIR REDUCTION WITH PULSED LIGHT

One of the early benefits of IPL was the observation of permanent hair reduction of dark hairs. Over the years, pulsed light has proved quite effective as a tool for safe and permanent hair reduction. The general principles for effective hair reduction with pulsed light are as follows. Dark hair responds; white hair does not. Two to 3 passes are more effective for hair reduction than a single pass, and higher number cutoff filters and higher fluences and longer pulse durations produce safe and effective hair reduction of dark terminal hairs in Fitzpatrick skin types I through IV. Because of the beneficial effect of pulsed light inflammatory lesions, pulsed light is especially effective for hair reduction, where pseudofolliculitis and inflammatory or hyperpigmentation are present.

Because of the effect on hair growth, an important consideration to take into account is when IPL is used where hair removal is not desired such as the beard area in men. To avoid undesired hair loss, it is recommended to either avoid treating areas where the patient does not desire to lose hair (eg, moustache or beard area) or to use very low fluences or small spot sizes to target lesions (vessels or pigmented lesions) in beard areas.

## DELAY OF SKIN AGING WITH PULSED LIGHT

One of the most important newer benefits of pulsed light treatments is the reported observations that regular treatments with pulsed light improve not only the appearance of aging skin but also skin appears to age more slowly. One of the early reports of the antiaging effects of pulsed light was reported in *Cutis* by the author and Dr Jason Pozner.[3] This retrospective photographic evaluation of 15 subjects receiving at least 1 and up to 4 BBL (Sciton Medical) treatments each year over an average of 9 years were judged by blinded evaluators to be the same age as their 9 -year-younger pretreatment photographs.

Other studies have confirmed the age-delaying effect of regular pulsed light treatments. In an interesting study looking at changes in gene expression of skin cells on forearm skin biopsies following 3 monthly treatments with BBL using a multiple-pass technique, Dr Chang, along with the author and colleagues from the Dermatology department at Stanford University School of Medicine, found nearly 1300 genes were "functionally" rejuvenated at 1 month after the last BBL treatment.[4] Key genes related to cell division, tumor suppression, and cell and organism longevity were rejuvenated to show messenger RNA levels similar to those found in skin biopsies of women in their twenties, even though the test subjects were aged 70 years.

The implications of the age-delaying effects of regular BBL treatments are profound and wide reaching. Patients now have the opportunity to not only keep their skin healthy but also keep their skin more youthful as they age. Skin anywhere on the body can benefit from the age-delaying effects of regular pulsed light treatments.

## WRINKLE REDUCTION, SKIN LAXITY, SKIN TIGHTENING TREATMENT WITH PULSED LIGHT

The observation of wrinkle reduction with pulsed light treatments is directly related to technique. The author has observed that the greatest skin texture improvements with pulsed light correlate with the greater number of pulses and passes performed at each treatment.

In general, fine wrinkles of the cheeks and crepey skin of the neck and fine wrinkles of sun-exposed skin improve the most. Wrinkles etched into the skin from repetitive muscle movement may also improve with repeated pulsed light treatments. Interestingly, wrinkle improvement seems to be correlated with more passes, regardless of the fluence or cutoff filter.

Delivery of pulsed light using a continual pulse mode is available on some IPL devices. BBL (Sciton Medical) uses a continual sequential pulsing of 2 xenon flash lamps that allow delivery of a continual train of pulses over several seconds. When this mode is used with a continual motion technique and the 590-nm cutoff filter (red and infrared light) or 800-nm cutoff filter (infrared light only), gradual skin and soft tissues are gradually heated. Target temperatures range from 40°C to 42°C, and treatment duration is 2 to 6 minutes at each treatment site.

The process of using Broad Band Light for bulk heating of skin and soft tissues produces collagen contraction and some degree of new dermal collagen formation. Both collagen contraction and neocollagenases can result in a modest degree of visible skin tightening. Typical treatment areas are cheeks, submentum, lower lids, infrabrow, and neck. Results seem to be technique dependent with better results achieved when target temperatures are sustained for up to 4 minutes. Results may last for 2 to 4 months after 1 to 4 treatments.

## ADJUNCTIVE BENEFITS OF PULSED LIGHT

There are several beneficial adjunctive uses of pulsed light. The benefits for improving postsurgical scarring early in the course of wound healing have been previously discussed. Pulsed light can be used to more quickly resolve procedure purpura and ecchymosis.

Purpura following injections can be performed the day after injections for any kind of filler or neuromodulator without concerns of diminishing the effect of the neuromodulator or correction and longevity of the filler.

Parameters are similar to those used for rosacea and scars. General guidelines are the darker the bruise, the lower the fluence. Dark ecchymosis or hematosis presents a large amount of extravasated hemoglobin as a target to the light. A parameter with a fluence that is too high can produce excessive heat that could result in a thermal burn. Many times a single pulsed light treatment over an ecchymosis can reduce the visible bruise effect 50% in 12 to 24 hours.

Pulsed light for swelling ecchymosis following a facelift procedure is best delayed for at least 2 weeks after the surgery to allow wound healing and reduction of swelling.

Pulsed light is an effective adjunctive treatment to resolve postablative laser erythema or postinflammatory hyperpigmentation. The author recommends waiting 2 to 3 weeks after full laser ablation and 7 to 10 days after fractionated laser before doing a pulsed light treatment. Parameters are the same as erythema and scarring, although the greater the postlaser erythema, the more conservative the practitioner should be with the fluence. A general principle is to reduce the fluence 2 J below typical parameters used for scars for the first treatment. Pulsed light treatments can be done every 2 to 3 weeks until erythema is resolved.

## FUTURE BENEFITS AND USES OF PULSED LIGHT

Areas where pulsed light may prove to have greater or preventative benefits in the future are possible skin cancer prevention, general body antiaging, and noninvasive body contouring and localized noninvasive fat reduction. Although early anecdotal observation has suggested reduced nonmelanoma skin cancer incidence in people receiving regular pulsed light treatments, these potential benefits need further study.

Systemic anti-aging from pulsed light treatments is conceivable considering the already demonstrated anti-aging effects on skin. Pulsed light devices deliver large fluences of red and infrared light that penetrate several centimeters beneath the skin surface deep into soft tissue and underlying vasculature. The effects of exposing blood circulating through the subcutaneous vascular plexus to visible and infrared light is not yet known. Future studies may show some anti-aging and health benefits that extend far beyond the benefits to skin.

Non-invasive fate reduction and body contouring are also conceivable considering the large amount of light energy in the red and infrared spectrum that is able to penetrate into subcutaneous fat heating large areas to temperatures that can begin to disrupt fat cells. Future studies to delineate the optimal parameters and treatment protocols will likely confirm pulsed light as an effective adjunctive treatment of fat reduction and body contouring.

## SUMMARY

Over the past 25 years, broad spectrum pulsed light has established its place in aesthetics and laser medicine. Pulsed light has proven its usefulness, effectiveness, and versatility in treating a multitude of skin problems, delaying skin aging, maintaining healthy skin, and as an adjunct to a cosmetic surgical practice in the treatment of postsurgical scars.

Practitioners contemplating adding a pulsed light device to their practice should choose a device that has at least 4 important features: (1) a large spot size; (2) variable-sized smaller spot adaptors; (3) pulse rates of at least 1 pulse per second; (4) a wide range of cutoff filters, including 515 nm, 560 nm, 590 nm, 640 nm, and 695 nm, to treat most skin types.

In addition, most practitioners should seek the best training by an experienced physician pulsed light practitioner. Training should cover the various applications of pulsed light, techniques, and parameters specific to each pulsed light device. Training should also cover prevention and management of pulsed light complications. If treatments are delegated to nonphysicians, each provider should receive the same thorough training before using pulsed light. Contrary to some technologies and devices introduced in the last 20 years, BBL will continue to be one of the major energy devices of laser and aesthetic practices.

The future of BBL is very bright as new technology and innovations make current treatments faster, more effective, and more cost-effective and continue to drive the discovery of a variety of new applications.

## DISCLOSURE

None.

## REFERENCES

1. Bitter PH Jr. Noninvasive rejuvenation of photodamaged skin using serial, full-face intense pulsed light treatments. Dermatol Surg 2000;26:835–43.

2. Bitter P Jr. Acne treatment with 3-step broadband light protocol. J Drugs Dermatol 2016;15(11):1382–8.

3. Bitter P Jr, Pozner J. Retrospective evaluation of the long-term antiaging effects of BroadBand Light therapy. Cosmetic Dermatology 2013;(Feb):34–40.

4. Chang ALS, Bitter PH Jr, Qu K, et al. Rejuvenation of gene expression pattern of aged human skin by broadband light treatment: a pilot study. J Invest Dermatol 2013;133(2):394–402.

# Nonablative and Hybrid Fractional Laser Skin Rejuvenation

Benjamin Carl Marcus, MD

## KEYWORDS

• Facial rejuvenation • Nonablative laser • Hybrid laser • Skin resurfacing

## KEY POINTS

- Nonablative laser therapy has been an active part of laser medicine for the better part of 15 years.
- Although the initial desire was to deliver a patient treatment that could improve skin aging without the downtime, modern fractional laser therapy has a myriad of indications and uses.
- Newer hybrid technologies deliver on the highly sought after therapy with minimal downtime but real improvement.

## INTRODUCTION

The history of skin resurfacing is a long and fascinating tale. The desire for facial rejuvenation is as old as many recorded histories. In ancient times, the Egyptians used sour milk to perform facial peels with the associated lactic acid.[1] Since those early days, there has been a long period of experimentation with different treatments to achieve the ideal balance between skin improvement and possible skin damage. In the modern era, there have already been several cycles of technological change. In the late 1980s to the mid 1990s, $CO_2$ laser dominated as the treatment of choice. Although this technique provided a robust improvement in skin texture, it carried with it a level of possible complications that some providers and many patients found to be too excessive.

In the early to mid 2000s, there was a significant expansion in technology that was described as "nonablative." These devices featured several different wavelengths and technologies. What they shared in common was the goal of delivering improvement in skin appearance while trying to minimize downtime and complications. Most of the "less-invasive" devices relied on the advent of fractional technology. This was the design feat of having multiple very small laser pulses delivered in a gridlike fashion. This allowed for a mosaic of treated and untreated skin. With islands of healthy skin next to treated skin, the healing process was thought to be more rapid.

Many of the wavelengths that were chosen for devices initially were selected to be nonablative. This meant that the laser did not induce true tissue vaporization. A very popular technology was the 1540-nm Erbium glass lasers. This technology produced columns of injured tissue but did not create channels of full tissue ablation. The author used this laser extensively in the early 2000s. Like many of these similar technologies, the patient tolerated the treatments very well. Long-term evaluation showed that results were modest.

Naturally, patients found the possible combination of limited downtime and moderate results to be very appealing. The trend culminated in the introduction of more powerful fractional laser devices. By the mid 2000s, the fractional technology was adapted to deliver microcolumns of ablative laser pulses. Some of the more popular devises featured fractionated $CO_2$ laser as well as Erbium:YAG (Er:YAG). Although these would normally be considered ablative devices when used in a full-field mode, when delivered in a fractionated

Disclosure Statement: The author has nothing to disclose.
University Hospital, 600 Highland Avenue, Madison, WI 53792, USA
*E-mail address:* marcus@surgery.wisc.edu

Facial Plast Surg Clin N Am 28 (2020) 37–44
https://doi.org/10.1016/j.fsc.2019.09.003

mode, they are classified as nonablative treatments.

The latest trend in this family of devices is the "hybrid" devices. These novel laser devices deliver a combination of more than 1 wavelength during the treatment. By combining fractionated but "ablative" wavelengths with true nonablative wavelengths, the physician has yet another tool in their toolbox to fit patients' specific needs.

## BACKGROUND

Laser terminology can be confusing. Technically, a nonablative laser works by releasing a coherent beam of light at a wavelength that is primarily absorbed by water. Naturally, with the target chromophore of water, this directly affects the cells of the skin. Depending on the particular wavelength used, the resultant energy transfer may cause only local tissue injury. This, in time, will produce columns of microtissue necrosis. Alternatively, a wavelength that is better absorbed by water can produce a true ablation. This leads to small columns of vaporization of the affected cells.

When looked at on a microscopic level, there is a distinct difference in these laser effects on skin cell architecture. Despite this, the fractionated lasers are generally grouped together under the category of nonablative. This is done, in effect, to differentiate them from ablative lasers that are used in a full-field fashion. Although they are semantic in nature, the distinction is important when considering treatment options. Full-field treatments (although very effective) produce a very different profile of healing time, risk, and outcome. Thus, a $CO_2$ laser when used in fractionated mode is often considered "nonablative." The same wavelength of laser when used in a full field mode is considered ablative.

## CLASSIC USES

In this section, the author reviews the established devices that have a solid track record and maintains an important part of the laser surgeon's armamentarium.

### Erbium Glass (1540 nm)

The Erbium glass laser has been available for several years. Their earliest history in evaluation goes back to the early 1980s.[2] The device became popular in the early 2000s. Part of the early appeal of these lasers was their ability to be used in multiple skin types. Because of the wavelength used, there was much less collateral damage to surrounding structures, such as melanocytes.

Early studies[3] with the device were able to demonstrate that the treatment could produce improvements in skin texture and quality. The unique aspect of this particular study was the use of ultrasound analysis. This thoughtful outcome measure was able to demonstrate a statistically significant improvement in the thickness of the treated dermis. One can conclude that this would be consistent with neocollagen production.

One of the popular current uses for Erbium glass lasers is the treatment of melasma. This laser is especially useful because the low profile of energy transfer makes melasma activation much less likely. A split face evaluation demonstrated that the Erbium glass laser can produce significant improvement in melasma with a very low-risk profile.[4] This study was limited to skin types that were a Fitzpatrick 3 or less. The author has used this device in patients with the full range of darker skin types. **Fig. 1** demonstrates long-term improvements in this patient with chronic hyperpigmentation and Fitzpatrick 5/6 skin.

A new and potentially useful application of the wavelength is in the treatment of stubborn striae or "stretch marks." This particular skin condition can occur after weight shift or body changes associated with pregnancy. This has long been a difficult condition to treat. Erbium glass is well tolerated and appropriate for the multiple sessions required. A study from 2016 showed that significant clinical improvement was observed after 6 sessions.[5] Histopathology was obtained and further ratified these results. With this in mind, those with this device may have a new use for this venerable technology.

### YSSG (2790 nm)

The yttrium, scandium, gallium and garnet (YSSG) laser was a star in the world of nonablative technology. It had a fairly similar profile for downtime as the Erbium glass laser. Because of its wavelength, the technology was able to produce even more significant energy transfer to the skin but without any real increase in risk to the patient.

Initial studies demonstrated that the technology was able to induce collagen, penetrate to a good depth within the dermis, and did not induce postinflammatory pigmentation.[6] Additional studies pursued the treatment endpoint farther.[7] As follow up stretched beyond two years better data became available. Although the improvement that patients saw at 6 weeks was outstanding for facial pigment and moderate for skin wrinkles, the improvement appeared to have a long duration. Patient evaluation shows that at 2 years after treatment, patients had an average of 57% of their initial improvement.

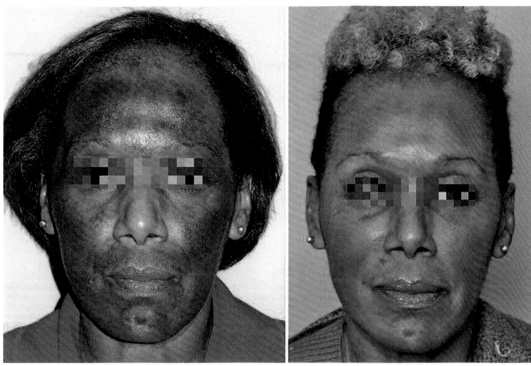

**Fig. 1.** A 56-year-old woman with Fitzpatrick type 5 skin. Severe dyschromias treated with multiple sessions of 1540-nm ER:glass laser.

Although this device appeared to have some real potential, it faded from practitioners use because of the promulgation of the new Er:YAG devices. There are limited studies available after 2013.

### Fractionated Erbium (2940 nm)

Fractional Er:YAG resurfacing has become of the mainstay of current nonablative treatment. There are a myriad of uses for this technology. Similar to other wavelengths discussed herein, the laser has water as its chromophore. As the wavelength with the best affinity for water, most energy is transferred with the pulse. At the same time, there is the least amount of collateral heat transfer. The bottom line of this configuration is that the Er:YAG pulses are nearly pure ablation. The absence of collateral heat transfer allows the device to produce deep ablation into the channels without damage to melanocytes.

An essential use of the Er:YAG fractional laser is rejuvenation of the skin and reduction of facial wrinkles. **Fig. 2** demonstrates a male patient who underwent 4 sessions of nonablative Er:YAG resurfacing. Initial healing is significantly diminished in these types of treatments. While the changes in aging skin are not as profound as in full face treatments with wide field ablative devices; the results are tangible and give real improvement for patients if adequate sessions are performed.

A valuable use for laser resurfacing is in the reduction of facial scars. The Er:YAG laser has solid backing as a useful modality.[8] The ability to have columns of pure ablation allows the operator to pursue significant depth (up to 600 μm in some cases). This depth has the ability to truly break up scar tissue and allows the ingrowth of healthy cells over time. **Fig. 3** shows a patient who had a motor vehicle accident. Her posttraumatic scar had been optimized with surgical revision. She then underwent a series of Er:YAG fractionated treatments. A significant improvement in her already mature scar is easily recognized.

Atrophic acne scars also have been shown to respond well to the pure ablative quality of the wavelength. **Fig. 4** demonstrates the results of 3 sessions of Er:YAG facial resurfacing with depth of penetration up to 500 μm. This type of clinical result is confirmed by the work of Sobanko and colleagues.[9] With sessions ranging from 3 to 6 repetitions, patients were able to appreciate significant improvement in their atrophic acne scars. Using 3-dimensional topographic modeling, estimates of efficacy ranged from 25% to 75%. There was much individual variation.

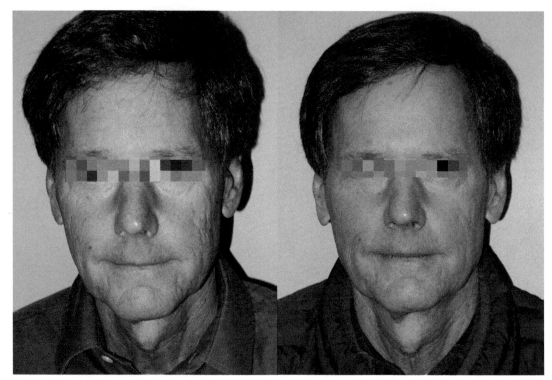

**Fig. 2.** A man with concerns for facial aging. He underwent 4 sessions of fractionated Erbium laser with good long-term improvements.

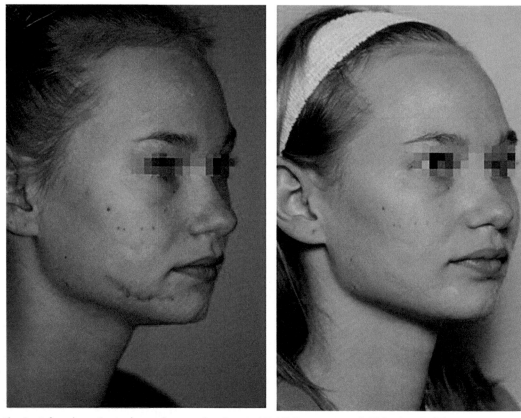

**Fig. 3.** A female patient who underwent fractionated Er:YAG treatments (×5) for her facial scar.

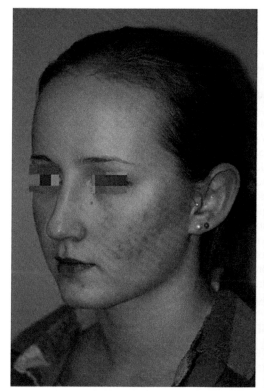 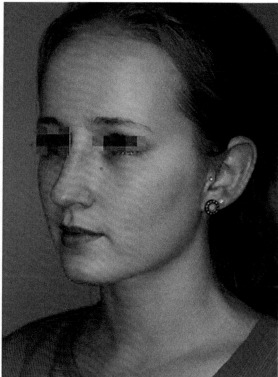

**Fig. 4.** A female patient who underwent fractioned Er:YAG treatments (×5) for her acne scars.

The natural presumption would be that if the Er:YAG is quite good at ablation without coagulation, then the fractionated $CO_2$ laser would be ideal for reduction of facial wrinkles. More coagulation should produce more collagen. A very interesting study recently demonstrated that although both technologies performed well with facial wrinkles reduction, there was no statistical difference between the 2.[10] With this information, it is fair to consider the Er:YAG laser as a very capable device for nonablative resurfacing in addition to scar improvement. A metaanalysis was also performed in 2018.[11] In this investigation, the focus was on comparison between fractionated $CO_2$ versus Er:YAG. Once again, there was not a major difference between the 2 in their outcome measures. They were both rated as much more effective than more standard Nd:YAG lasers.

### Fractioned $CO_2$ (10,000 nm)

The main functional difference with the fractionated $CO_2$ lasers when compared with the Er:YAG lasers centers on the wavelengths themselves. With a higher amount of collateral heat transfer, the fractionated $CO_2$ laser is much more likely to produce a collagen response (in theory). Although this would be a good thing, the potential success is mitigated by the inability to treat Fitzpatrick

skin scores greater than 3. Er:YAG, on the other hand, can be used all the way through Fitzpatrick 6.

As cited above, most studies that do a split face or head-to-head treatment show that the 2 treatments produce very similar results. Therefore, when would it be advisable for a provider to choose Er:YAG over $CO_2$? The main consideration would be the likelihood to need to treat darker skin types. In a practice that encounters more Fitzpatrick scores 3 and above, the Er:YAG device will have the greatest versatility.

Although there is no definitive study that indicates superiority for the fractionated $CO_2$ device, there are several studies that demonstrate efficacy and/or equivalency. The devices have been helpful in reduction of striae,[12] scars,[13] facial wrinkles, and burns.[14]

### CURRENT TRENDS

In this section, the newer devices that have shown a potential to be valuable to the laser surgeons armamentarium are reviewed. This group of devices intends to improve the degree of facial rejuvenation by stacking carefully selected wavelength dyads. By having energy delivered by different wavelengths at the same time, there can be a greater amount of energy delivered to different stratifications of the skin architecture.

## Halo

The "Halo" device is proprietary to Sciton (Palo Alto, CA, USA). This device combines a traditional Er:YAG fractional laser and is crafted to codeliver a second simultaneous pulse of laser light at 1470 nm. The "noninvasive" wavelength at 1470 nm can be programmed to go quite deep. This insures collagen stimulation without dramatic skin recovery. The addition of a traditional microablation laser ensures that the upper layers of skin are improved in the arenas of pigment production, and overall rejuvenation is still a "weekend" style of recovery.

The initial study[15] that evaluated this technology demonstrated some interesting findings. Most patients felt that they had minimal pain from the procedure. It was made to be done under a topical anesthetic without oral pain medication. Blinded photographic analysis led to an 80% rate for "significant" improvement. Perhaps the most telling statistic was the 100% patient satisfaction. A total of 34 female patients were treated in the study. One element that was particularly well rated was the effect on dyschromias. There have not been further major studies on the device, but the efficacy was deemed good enough that the device was given a Food and Drug Administration indication for melasma. With melasma being one of the more difficult conditions to treat, this is a welcome addition.

One of the more popular trends in laser medicine right now is the concept of "prejuvenation." Many younger patients will present with a desire to improve, but more importantly, preserve their skin. Often a combination therapy with an intense pulsed light device and the hybrid fractional device (HALO) is offered. This combination of treatment offers very modest to minimal downtime and good clinical outcomes. Long-range studies with this configuration are needed, but it is an exciting area and a treatment plan that is quite promising. **Fig. 5** demonstrates a patient who has undergone 3 sessions with the hybrid fractional HALO device.

## SPECIAL CONSIDERATIONS

Technology in the world of laser medicine moves very quickly. There are several novel uses and indications for fractional laser therapy. One of the more exciting future directions is drug delivery.

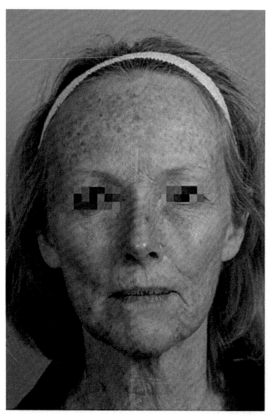 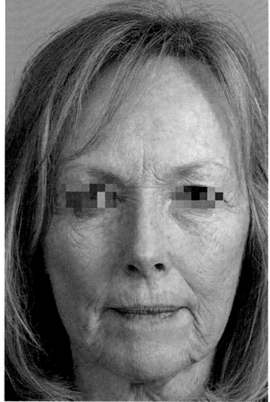

**Fig. 5.** A patient before and after 3 sessions with the HALO device.

By creating channels in the skin, either modality of $CO_2$ or Er:YAG has the ability to facilitate the localization of drugs to the intradermal space. There are great implications for this, including magnifying the effect of rejuvination techniques or facilitating the treatment of skin conditions.

For rejuvenation, laser-assisted drug delivery has been shown to be helpful for several conditions. Research from 2018 showed an improvement in hair regrowth when scalp tissue was pretreated with fractional laser and Finasteride was delivered to the scalp.[16] Other studies have tried to synergize the rejuvenation from the laser with biochemical actions of bioactive compounds. Application of the patient's own platelet-rich plasma has been investigated and found to have a positive outcome when compared with laser alone.[17]

Laser-assisted drug delivery has been evaluated in the context of treating skin cancers. Although topical 5 flouro-uracil has been used for quite some time, a study in 2015 demonstrated that the drug penetration would be enhanced with pretreatment with the fractionated $CO_2$ device.[18]

In addition to drug delivery, fractional laser therapy has been evaluated to see if it could play a role in decreasing skin cancers before they fully present. Although there are no definitive studies in humans, there have been positive data to come out of an animal study in 2015.[19] This novel study showed a reduction in the formation of skin cancers in a mouse model whereby there was UV exposure. When compared with the cohort without laser treatment, they had statistically fewer skin cancers form.

## SUMMARY

Nonablative laser therapy has been an active part of laser medicine for the better part of 15 years. Although the initial desire was to deliver a patient treatment that could improve skin aging without the downtime, modern fractional laser therapy has a myriad of indications and uses. Newer hybrid technologies deliver on the highly sought after therapy with minimal downtime but real improvement. Stronger more traditional fractional devices have great utility in the area of scar improvement, major pigment removal, and even drug delivery.

Although there is no device that can truly delivery exceptional skin rejuvenation without a degree of downtime, the current array of fractional laser still plays a key and critical role for the laser medicine specialist who needs to treat a variety of conditions, skin types, and expectations.

## REFERENCES

1. The secret of ancient Egyptian beauty. Arab News 2019.
2. Gaponstev VP, Matitsin AA, Kravchenko VB. Erbium glass lasers and their applications. Opt Laser Technol 1982;14(4):189–96.
3. Dahan S, Lagarde JM, Turlier V, et al. Treatment of neck lines and forehead rhytids with a nonablative 1540-nm Er:glass laser: a controlled clinical study combined with the measurement of the thickness and the mechanical properties of the skin. Dermatol Surg 2004;30(6):872–9.
4. Barysch MJ, Rümmelein B, Kolm I, et al. Split-face study of melasma patients treated with non-ablative fractionated photothermolysis (1540nm). J Eur Acad Dermatol Venereol 2012;26(4):423–30.
5. Wang K, Ross N, Osley K, et al. Evaluation of a 1540-nm and a 1410-nm nonablative fractionated laser for the treatment of striae. Dermatol Surg 2016;42(2):225–31.
6. Ross EV, Swann M, Soon S, et al. Full-face treatments with the 2790-nm erbium:YSGG laser system. J Drugs Dermatol 2009;8(3):248–52.
7. Walgrave SE, Kist DA, Noyaner-Turley A, et al. Minimally ablative resurfacing with the confluent 2,790 nm erbium:YSGG laser: a pilot study on safety and efficacy. Lasers Surg Med 2012;44(2):103–11.
8. Kim SG, Kim EY, Kim YJ, et al. The efficacy and safety of ablative fractional resurfacing using a 2,940-Nm Er:YAG laser for traumatic scars in the early posttraumatic period. Arch Plast Surg 2012;39(3):232–7.
9. Sobanko JF, Alster TS. Management of acne scarring, part I: a comparative review of laser surgical approaches. Am J Clin Dermatol 2012;13(5):319–30.
10. Robati RM, Asadi E. Efficacy and safety of fractional $CO_2$ laser versus fractional Er:YAG laser in the treatment of facial skin wrinkles. Lasers Med Sci 2017;32(2):283–9.
11. Ansari F, Sadeghi-Ghyassi F, Yaaghoobian B. The clinical effectiveness and cost-effectiveness of fractional $CO_2$ laser in acne scars and skin rejuvenation: a meta-analysis and economic evaluation. J Cosmet Laser Ther 2018;20(4):248–51.
12. Soliman M, Mohsen Soliman M, El-Tawdy A, et al. Efficacy of fractional carbon dioxide laser versus microneedling in the treatment of striae distensae. J Cosmet Laser Ther 2019;21(5):270–7.
13. Zhang Y, Liu Y, Cai B, et al. Improvement of surgical scars by early intervention with carbon dioxide fractional laser. Lasers Surg Med 2019. [Epub ahead of print].
14. Douglas H, Lynch J, Harms KA, et al. Carbon dioxide laser treatment in burn-related scarring: a

prospective randomised controlled trial. J Plast Reconstr Aesthet Surg 2019;72(6):863–70.

15. Waibel S, Pozner J, Robb C, et al. Hybrid fractional laser: a multi-center trial on the safety and efficacy for photorejuvenation. J Drugs Dermatol 2018; 17(11):1164–8.

16. Bertin ACJ, Vilarinho A, Junqueira ALA. Fractional non-ablative laser-assisted drug delivery leads to improvement in male and female pattern hair loss. J Cosmet Laser Ther 2018;20(7–8):391–4.

17. Araco A. A prospective study comparing topic platelet-rich plasma vs. placebo on reducing superficial perioral wrinkles and restore dermal matrix. J Cosmet Laser Ther 2019;1–7. [Epub ahead of print].

18. Glenn CJ, Parlette EC, Mitchell C. Fractionated $CO_2$ laser-assisted delivery of topical 5-fluorouracil as a useful modality for treating field cutaneous squamous cell carcinomas. Dermatol Surg 2015;41(11): 1339–42.

19. Jagdeo JR, Brody NI, Spandau DF, et al. Important implications and new uses of ablative lasers in dermatology: fractional carbon dioxide laser prevention of skin cancer. Dermatol Surg 2015;41(3): 387–9.

# Chemical Peel (Deep, Medium, Light)

Sidney J. Starkman, MD[a], Devinder S. Mangat, MD[b],*

## KEYWORDS

- Chemical peel • Chemoexfoliation • Phenol-croton oil peel • Skin resurfacing

## KEY POINTS

- Chemical peels offer an excellent option for skin resurfacing for rhytids and dyschromias.
- Phenol-croton oil peels have been modernized dependent on croton oil concentration to minimize risks.
- Complications associated with chemical peels are uncommon with proper technique and postoperative management.

## INTRODUCTION

With modern medicine increasing both the average life span and quality of life, there has been a greater demand for treatment of age-related skin changes. This has led to a boon in skin care products, and medical devices. As many new options in skin resurfacing are developed annually, it is chemical peeling that has withstood the trials of time and scrutiny. Ever since 1550 BC when keratolytic formulas were mentioned in the Ebers Papyrus, and more recently with the laypeelers of the twentieth century, chemoexfoliation has been the standard by which other methods of skin resurfacing are measured.

The different variations of chemoexfoliation have been used for rhytids, actinic damage, lentigos, and dyschromias. The goal of this article was to describe the most recent knowledge about chemical peeling, and to expose the previously accepted yet incorrect dogmas. Chemical peeling, when practiced with knowledge and good technique, can yield excellent results in skin rejuvenation.

## HISTORY

Before becoming common practice of plastic surgeons, chemical peeling was modernized via the laypeelers of the 1920s. In Hollywood, laypeelers would cater to the movie stars who wished to maintain youthful skin and facial features. Some of the foundational laypeelers of the twentieth century were Jean DeDesly and Antoinette LaGasse. The physicians began to incorporate chemical peeling into their practices in the 1950s and 1960s. There is a 4-part series by Gregory Hetter that details the transition of chemical peeling from the hands of the laypeelers to the plastic surgeons.

As chemoexfoliation entered the realm of medical practice and literature, the experiences of the many plastic surgeons became publicly described. Some writings were more scientific, and other publications were more anecdotal in nature. In some cases, dogma was written and followed for decades.

## PATIENT SELECTION

A critical portion of practicing chemical peeling is the identification of the suitable patient. The patient must both be a physical candidate for a chemical peel, and also have appropriate expectations for their postpeel results. Skin-related changes, such as rhytids and photodamage, must be distinguished from other changes like volume loss or jowling. Ideally, a chemical peel

[a] Facial Plastic Surgeon, Mangat Plastic Surgery, 56 Edwards Village Boulevard, Suite 226, Edwards, CO 81632, USA; [b] Starkman Facial Plastic Surgery, 8560 E Shea Boulevard, Suite 110, Scottsdale, AZ 85260, USA
* Corresponding author. 133 Barnwood Drive, Edgewood, KY.
E-mail address: devindermangat5@gmail.com

Facial Plast Surg Clin N Am 28 (2020) 45–57
https://doi.org/10.1016/j.fsc.2019.09.004

patient will have blue eyes, fair skin, and shallow rhytids. However, most chemical peel patients will not fit this exact description. Most commonly, the Fitzpatrick scale is used to help define a patient's skin type (**Table 1**).

Patients also can be rated by their skin type, texture, complexion, and photoaging, using categorizing schemes such as the one by Glogau (**Table 2**).

The medical history of the patient must be reviewed before any chemical peeling occurs. Relative contraindications for any resurfacing procedure include smoking, diabetes, active or frequent herpes simplex virus (HSV) infections, cutaneous radiation history, hypertrophic scarring, or keloid history. Photosensitizing drugs, exogenous estrogen, and birth control pills should be avoided because of the increased risk of hyperpigmentation. Patients also should be warned not to have plans to become pregnant within 6 months after chemical peeling, because of elevated estrogen levels of pregnancy.[1]

Smoking and sun exposure always should be addressed in the planning stages. Chemical peels on the faces of chronic smokers can lead to poor tissue healing, because of the microvascular damage from smoking. It is recommended that smokers stop 1 month before the peel and continue abstinence for at least 6 months afterward. Likewise, it should be recommended to patients that prolonged sun exposure should be avoided for 3 months after the peel. If this is unacceptable to the patient, other options besides chemical peeling should be explored.

An absolute contraindication to chemical peeling, or any facial resurfacing, is recent use of isotretinoin (Accutane). Isotretinoin prevents reepithelialization from hair follicles and sebaceous glands, and chemical peeling relies primarily on this reepithelialization for healing. The most current recommendations are to stop isotretinoin for 12 to 24 months before the peel.

Finally, the patient and the practitioner must have agreed on the reasonable expectations of the peel. The patient's axillary skin can represent the final result of the chemical peel, as long as this region has not previously received excessive sun damage.[2]

## PREPARATION

After the patient selection and planning are completed, adequate skin preparation must begin before the peel. Sunscreens should be started 3 months beforehand to prevent prepeel tanning or sunburns. Part of the purpose of this is to decrease the melanocyte activity before the peel. Topical tretinoin (Retin-A) is recommended for 6 to 12 weeks before the peel. The topical tretinoin has been shown to have a synergistic effect with trichloroacetic acid (TCA) peels, and can sustain the effects of these peels.[3–5] Tretinoin leads to exfoliation of stratum corneum and increased melanin distribution, and aids in proper penetration of the peel solution. The tretinoin contributes to a thickened and uniform epidermis, which aids in uniform application of the peeling agent.

Nighttime tretinoin treatments can begin 6 weeks before the peel, and continue until the postpeel reepithelialization is completed. The dosing ranges from 0.025% to 0.1%; however, no literature has shown improved results with the higher dosing. Patients should be counseled of the possible side effects of tretinoin, such as erythema, flakiness, or skin irritation. If this was to occur, the dose can be reduced or the medication can be discontinued entirely.

**Table 1**
**Fitzpatrick skin type scale**

| Skin Type | Skin Color | Characteristics |
| --- | --- | --- |
| I | White; very fair; red or blond hair; blue eyes; freckles | Always burns; never tans |
| II | White; fair; red or blond hair; blue, hazel, or green eyes | Usually burns, tans with difficulty |
| III | Cream white; fair with any eye or hair color; very common | Sometimes mild burn, gradually tans |
| IV | Brown; typical Mediterranean white skin | Rarely burns, tans with ease |
| V | Dark brown; Middle Eastern skin types | Very rarely burns, tans very easily |
| VI | Black | Nevers burns, tans very easily |

**Table 2**
**Glogau skin classification scale**

| Group I (Mild) | Group II (Moderate) | Group III (Advanced) | Group IV (Severe) |
|---|---|---|---|
| No keratoses | Early actinic keratoses-slight yellow skin discoloration | Actinic keratoses-obvious yellow skin discoloration with telangiectasias | Actinic keratoses and skin cancers have occurred |
| Little wrinkling | Early wrinkling-parallel skin lines | Wrinkling present at rest | Wrinkling: much cutis laxa of actinic, gravitational, and dynamic origin |
| No scarring | Mild scarring | Moderate acne scarring | Severe acne scarring |
| Little or no makeup | Little makeup | Wears makeup always | Wears makeup that cakes on |

Another beneficial drug in the preparation of chemical peel patients is hydroquinone. Hydroquinone is used mostly in patients with dyschromias or lentigos, or in patients with Fitzpatrick III, IV, V, and VI skin types, because of the elevated risks of postpeel postinflammatory hyperpigmentation. The mechanism of hydroquinone is to block the conversion of tyrosine to L-Dopa by tyrosinase, thereby decreasing melanin production. In applicable patients, hydroquinone in a concentration of 4% to 8% should be started 4 to 6 weeks before chemical peeling. Recommended formula for prepeel skin preparation is the following: hydroquinone 8%, hydrocortisone 1%, and Retin-A 0.05% in a moisturizing cream base. Similar to tretinoin, hydroquinone should be restarted after the peel once the patient's skin is ready to tolerate it. All patients should be warned of the possibility of HSV outbreaks, even if they deny any history of herpetic vesicle breakouts. It is possible to harbor latent infections even without any apparent clinical history. Recommended practice is to start any patient with a negative history on a prophylactic dose of antivirals, acyclovir 400 mg 3 times a day, 3 days before and continued for at least 7 days after the peel. For patients who do have a history of herpetic breakouts, a therapeutic dose of antivirals should be used, such as valacyclovir 1 g 3 times a day for the aforementioned time period.

The first line of resistance to bacterial infection is the skin, and resurfacing procedures can reduce this barrier. This can lead to infections by cutaneous bacterial flora, such as staphylococcal or streptococcal species. Appropriate antibacterial coverage should begin before the peel as prophylaxis. The senior author (DSM) uses cephalexin, 250 mg 4 times a day, 1 day before the peel and continues it for 7 days in the postoperative period. In patients who are B-lactam sensitive, erythromycin 250 mg 4 times a day can be used. To maintain uniform depth of the peeling agent, it is advisable to recommend avoiding microdermabrasion, waxing, or electrolysis for 3 to 4 weeks before peeling.

## DEFINING DEPTH OF PEEL

The depth of a chemical peel is characterized by the amount of penetration, amount of destruction of the epidermis and dermis, and inflammatory response. A superficial chemical peel is an appropriate option for patients with superficial lentigos, mild actinic damage, and fine rhytids. This has a much greater safety and fewer complications than deep chemical peels. The superficial peel penetrates through the entire epidermis and causes epidermal sloughing. It will also cause an inflammatory response in the upper portion of the papillary dermis. For patients with Glogau types III or IV classification and Fitzpatrick type I and II, a deep peel such as the classic Baker formulation can be used in the perioral area. Deep peels cause sloughing of the epidermis and papillary dermis, and inflammation of the reticular dermis. The deep peel is most effective in erasing deep rhytids, but it also carries the highest risk of complications, such as scarring with the 50% TCA peel or hypopigmentation with the classic Baker formula. With superficial and deep peels comprising 2 ends of the spectrum of chemical peeling, the medium-depth peel balances excellent results with low risks. The medium-depth peel effectively treats moderate photoaging skin (Glogau II), dyschromias, and mild-to-moderate acne scars.

## SUPERFICIAL PEELS

The workhorse peel for plastic surgeons, dermatologists, and aestheticians has been the alpha-hydroxy acids (AHAs). Various AHAs of differing types and strengths have made their way into over-the-counter skincare products. However, this wide application still requires that providers know the clinical characteristics and safety profile of these chemicals.

AHAs are natural fruit, carboxylic acids, with the most common AHA being glycolic acid or 2-hydroxyethanoic acid. Glycolic acid is derived from sugar cane and is generally used in a concentration of 20% to 70%. Other common AHAs are citric acid (2-hydroxyl 1,2,3 propanetricarboxylic acid), found in citrus fruit, and lactic acid (2-hydroxypropanoic acid), found in sour milk and tomato juice.[6] Salicylic acid, in concentrations of 20% to 30%, is also used in superficial chemical peels.

AHAs penetrate through the epidermis and the most superficial layer of the dermis. They work by diminishing the cohesion between the keratinocytes of the stratum granulosum. This leads to the sloughing of the abnormal cells and thins the stratum corneum. These benefits generally last for 2 to 3 weeks.

Although superficial chemical peels do have a high safety profile, a false sense of security should be avoided with AHAs. Without neutralization, glycolic acid can have persistent effects and penetrate deeply. Its action should be neutralized with water. If glycolic acid remains un-neutralized, the deeper penetration can lead to healing problems, crusting, and scarring. The anticipated endpoint of a glycolic acid peel should be erythema and light peeling of the epidermis.[7]

Jessner solution (14 g salicylic acid, 14 g lactic acid, and 14 g resorcinol in 100 mL of ethanol) is a superficial peeling agent with a high safety profile. The depth of penetration depends on the number of coats applied. If 1 to 3 coats are applied, exfoliation of the stratum corneum occurs. If 5 to 10 coats are applied, the depth of penetration continues down to the basal layer.

## DEEP PEELS

The peel relies on injury down to the reticular dermis to treat the deep rhytids of the lateral canthal and perioral regions. Although the papillary dermis is thought to heal via reorganization, the reticular dermis is thought to heal via scarring.[8] With deep chemical peeling, additional recovery time is necessary, and the risk of scarring is higher.

The workhorse deep chemical peel agent was the Baker-Gordon formulation; however, this lost some popularity as TCA peels and $CO_2$ laser surfacing rose into the field. The Baker-Gordon peel did offer arguably unparalleled treatment for deep facial rhytids, but the irreversible hypopigmentation risk and the cardiac/renal toxicity limited its applicability.

Another option for deep peels is the 50% TCA peel; however, a significant percentage of patients develop scarring with this formulation. This catastrophic complication halted the application of this strength of TCA solution.

Notwithstanding the risks of the Baker-Gordon peel, it does have a role in the correct scenario. In patients with deepened rhytids in distinct facial subunits with Fitzpatrick I and II skin types, this is a very effective peeling option. Nonetheless, a high level of technique and caution must be used to avoid excessively deep peeling with this solution. A uniform application of peeling solution with mindfulness of the developing frost will help to prevent potential complications.

## MEDIUM-DEPTH PEELS

Current discussion and development of modern-day chemical peel centers around the medium-depth peeling agents. Medium-depth peels penetrate through the epidermis and the papillary dermis and cause some inflammation in the upper reticular dermis. The standard medium peel has been the 35% TCA peel. It does not have systemic toxicities, and it is very easy to store, as it does not require refrigeration in its crystalline form. However, the risk of scarring with TCA is much higher than with phenol-based peeling solutions. TCA solution concentrations are measured strictly on weight by volume (grams per 100 mL distilled water). Any miscommunication between the provider and the pharmacy in the manner of mixing the TCA solution would be catastrophic. TCA concentrations of 50% or more greatly increase the possibility of scarring.[9] There have been no additional techniques that have proven beneficial in reducing this risk of scarring.[10]

To achieve medium-depth peels without the risks of scarring, providers have been combining 35% TCA solutions with other less potent agents. The additional solution is applied first as an epidermolytic, and this enhances the depth of penetration of the 35% TCA peel solution. This technique was first described by Brody, using $CO_2$ ice and acetone to create epidermal break for the TCA solution that follows.[11]

Another combination peel is Jessner solution followed by 35% TCA, described by Monheit.[12] Jessner solution plays the role of penetrating the epidermis, and TCA is then applied once the

Jessner solution has dried.[12] Unlike with phenol peels, frosting does not occur immediately, and 3 to 4 minutes must be allowed for the full frost to form. Once this has happened, additional coats can be applied to reach the desired depth of peel. Care is taken with additional applications of TCA, as this has a cumulative effect and leads to a deeper peel, thus increasing the changes of hypopigmentation and scarring.

Coleman and Futrell[13] experimented with creating a combination peel out of glycolic acid and 35% TCA. Their histologic examinations demonstrated that it penetrated slightly deeper than Jessner/TCA combination peels.[13]

Investigations by Brody[11] into the complications of these 3 combination peels found that their risks of scarring were less than 1%. This scarring risk placed them on par with other skin resurfacing modalities, such as phenol-croton oil peels or $CO_2$ laser resurfacing.

## MODIFIED PHENOL-CROTON OIL PEELS

TCA peel solutions have taken a prominent role in modern-day chemical peel practices, due to the all-or-none qualities of the Baker-Gordon phenol-croton oil peel. Decades-worth of anecdotal experiences regarding phenol-croton oil peels made their way into the literature. The descriptions began in the 1950s and 1960s when plastic surgeons first adopted the phenol-croton oil solutions. Litton[14] was the first to present these formulas to the American Society of Plastic and Reconstructive Surgery in the late 1950s. Soon afterward, the classic formula was credited to Baker in the early 1960s.[15]

Around this time in the 1960s, Adolph Brown[16] wrote extensively about phenol-croton oil peels. He presented 3 doctrines of phenol peeling. First, increasing the concentration of phenol (80% to 90%) would work to prevent further penetration by creating an immediate keratocoagulation. Second, adding a saponin to the solution would increase the depth of penetration. Third, the role of croton oil was merely to buffer the solution. These writings were accepted as standards, and additionally felt that phenol was the sole active ingredient within the Baker formula. This resulted in the belief that phenol in lower concentrations was more dangerous because of deeper penetration and that croton oil had no role in the depth of peel. These beliefs lasted until the 1990s, when they were questioned by Gregory Hetter.[15]

Croton oil is pressed from the seeds of Croton tiglium, a small shrub found in India and Ceylon. Croton oil comprises mostly oleic, myristic, arachidonic, and linoleic acids. In 1935, Joseph R. Spies[17] discovered that croton oil was soluble in ethanol and benzene, but poorly soluble in a 50:50 mixture of phenol to water. Hetter[15] theorized that this may be why septisol is needed as a surfactant in the Baker formula.

Hetter[15] investigated the role of croton oil and phenol in chemoexfoliation by experimenting on a volunteer with multiple formulations of varying concentrations of phenol and croton oil. These experiments refuted the previously described dogmas of the mid-twentieth century. A solution of 18% phenol without croton oil demonstrated minimal postpeel effect. With a 35% phenol solution, mild keratolysis occurred with no dermal effect. It was only with an 88% phenol solution that a papillary dermal effect took place. When croton oil was added to the phenol solution, more substantial postpeel effects were noticed. In addition, varying croton oil concentrations had different results. A 0.7% croton oil concentration solution required a 7-day recovery period, whereas a 2.1% croton oil concentration required an 11-day recovery period. Hetter[15] thus postulated that higher concentrations of phenol (88%) without septisol would peel more deeply than lower concentrations (50% and 35%). He also remarked that phenol formulations result in deeper peels with increasing concentrations of croton oil.

Hetter's subsequent studies allowed him to form scientific generalizations in regard to phenol-croton oil chemical peels. He realized that by diluting the concentration of croton oil in these formulas, the healing times would be shortened, signifying a shallower depth of penetration. He took these assertions further by stating that the concentration of phenol in fact had little to do with the depth of penetration. Obagi[18] was the first to suggest that different concentrations of these formulas should be applied to the discrete subunits of the face (**Fig. 1**). Hetter used this postulation to apply varying concentrations of croton oil to the facial subunits. He found that the lower nose could tolerate croton oil concentrations up to 1.2%; the cheeks and forehead only tolerated concentrations up to 0.8%; and the upper nose, temple, and lateral brow could only withstand concentrations up to 0.4% before the risk of complications rose. Last, Hetter felt 1% croton oil solutions were the upper threshold for safe use to avoid serious risk of hypopigmentation.

Hetter first created his formulations using phenol at 33% to carry croton oil at 1-drop (0.35%), 2-drop (0.7%), and 3-drop (1.1%) concentrations. However, he soon switched to a more standardized system of measurement, rather

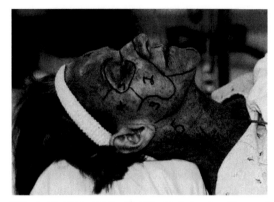

**Fig. 1.** Varying areas of skin texture, quality, and thickness marking the concentration of peeling agent to be used.

than relying on a dropper, which is naturally unreliable. He converted 1 drop into 1 cubic centimeter, and used this conversion to make a stock solution of 0.04 mL of croton oil per 1 mL of phenol. From this, he could make different croton oil formulations of 0.4%, 0.8%, 1.2%, and 1.6% in a constant phenol concentration (**Table 3**).

## TECHNIQUE

Before application of the peeling solution, the skin must be sufficiently prepared. This starts with a vigorous cleaning with septisol or acne wash the evening before and the morning of the chemical peel. Preoperative oral sedation, 10 mg diazepam and 100 mg dimenhydrinate (Dramamine), help to relieve patient anxiety. The antihistamine serves to reduce oral secretions and protect the patient's airway during the sedation. Intravenous fluids should be started before bringing the patient to the procedure room, as the patient will have had nothing to drink since the previous night.

Preoperative marking consists of marking the patient's submandibular shadow while in the

upright position. This serves to avoid noticeable delineation between the peeled and unpeeled areas of the neck. The patient is then placed in the supine position.

After appropriate sedation has been reached, supraorbital, infraorbital, and mental nerve blocks are performed with a 50:50 mixture of 2% lidocaine and 0.5% bupivacaine. Local anesthetic is also applied via a field block over the areas to be peeled. Epinephrine is avoided, as this will slow the clearance of the phenol. The face is meticulously degreased with an acetone-soaked gauze. Residual skin oil on the patient's face will impair the uniform application of the peeling agent. Other investigators, such as Hetter and Obagi, suggest using a wrung-out 2-inch × 2-inch gauze for the application of the peeling agent; however, the senior author feels that using a wide cotton-tipped applicator allows for superior control of application.

A benefit of phenol-based chemical peels is the frosting occurs almost immediately, as opposed to TCA where the frost can take 3 to 4 minutes to occur. This means that the quality and uniformity of depth, and need for reapplication, is almost immediately clear to the provider in a phenol-based peel. Medium-depth peels should result in a level II to level III frost (**Fig. 2**).[19,20]

Level I: erythema with stringy or blotchy frosting
Level II: white-coat with erythema showing through (should be used for eyelids and areas of bony prominences, that is, zygomatic arch, malar, chin… higher rate of scarring)

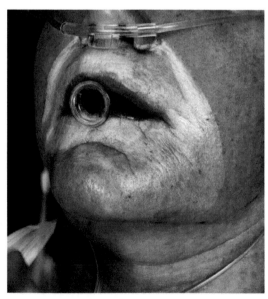

**Fig. 2.** A level 3 frost obtained during phenol-croton oil peeling in the perioral region.

| Table 3 Hetter peel formulations (stock solution = 24 mL + 1 mL croton oil [4% croton oil]) | | | | | |
|---|---|---|---|---|---|
| Croton oil, % | 0.2 | 0.4 | 0.8 | 1.2 | 1.6 |
| Distilled water, mL | 5.5 | 5.5 | 5.5 | 5.5 | 5.5 |
| Septisol, mL | 0.5 | 0.5 | 0.5 | 0.5 | 0.5 |
| USP Phenol 88%, mL | 3.5 | 3.0 | 2.0 | 1.0 | 0 |
| Stock solution containing phenol and croton oil, mL | 0.5 | 1.0 | 2.0 | 3.0 | 4.0 |
| Total, mL | 10 | 10 | 10 | 10 | 10 |

Level III: solid white frost with little or no background erythema

The facial subunits are divided by the severity of rhytids, photodamage, and lentigos, as well as skin thickness. The senior author uses 0.8% croton oil Hetter solution in areas of thicker skin and deeper rhytids (Glogau III and IV), such as the glabella and perioral regions. Intermediate areas (Glogau II and III) are treated with 0.4% croton oil Hetter solution. An 89% phenol solution is used for feathering along the borders of the peeled areas to achieve an even postpeel result. A classic Baker formula can be used in patients who are Fitzpatrick types I or II, and have severe Glogau IV rhytids in the upper lip.

Ten to 15 minutes are allowed between each subunit peeled for adequate clearance of the phenol. Less clearance time is needed with the Hetter solution because of lower phenol compared with the Baker-Gordon peel. The entire face can be peeled over 30 to 60 minutes. In the case that a minor supraventricular arrhythmia occurs, the peel should be paused until the patient returns to normal sinus rhythm.

When applying the peeling solution to the forehead and temporal regions, the peel should continue up to and even into the hairline. Phenol and croton oil will not affect the pigment of the hair follicles. In addition, in the perioral area, the peel should continue just over the vermilion border. This is because the margin of each peeled region will have a distinct line of reactive hyperemia. While peeling adjacent facial subunits, these lines of hyperemia should be included and peeled to prevent any resultant lines of demarcation. For deep wrinkles of the perioral region, the skin can be stretched taut to evenly apply the peel to these rhytids. Phenol-croton oil peels do not need to be neutralized, like glycolic acid peels, due to the completed reaction, as demonstrated by the frost.

An area to exercise caution is in the lower eyelid region. The phenol-croton oil peel should be applied to within 3 mm of the lower eyelid margin and then stopped. The sedated patient can develop tearing during the peeling procedure, and these tears should be wiped away to prevent the peeling solution from tracking up along the tear into the eye. The peel solution is not applied to the upper eyelid skin, as this area lacks the sebaceous glands that are necessary for reepithelialization after a peel.

If there were any areas of inadequate local anesthesia, the patient can experience an immediate burning sensation on application of the peeling solution, which will last for approximately 15 to 30 seconds. The burning sensation can then return approximately 30 minutes later and can last for the remainder of the procedure day. The bupivacaine in the local anesthetic blocks should provide anesthesia for hours following the peel. This is part of the reason why it is critical to apply comprehensive local anesthetic blocks to the peeled areas.

## POSTOPERATIVE PERIOD

The postoperative period begins immediately after the final subunit of the face is peeled. Once the last area of frosting dissipates and only erythema remains, a thick coat of emollient is applied to all of the peeled skin areas. The senior author prefers to use Eucerin cream, but Elta or Bacitracin ointment are other acceptable alternatives. These emollients are not occlusive and therefore do not affect the depth of the peel. The patient is instructed to maintain a steady coat of this emollient over the entire peeled region by reapplying 4 to 5 times per day, or as often as needed. This is continued for the duration of the postpeel period until the area has fully peeled, and fresh skin is visible.

The provider and staff should adequately explain the expectations for the immediate postpeel period to the patient. The patient's preoperative understanding of the expected burning sensation in the immediate postpeel will help with his or her tolerance. The patient also should be prescribed an oral narcotic. In addition, the patient should be prepared for the expected erythema, edema, and gradual desquamation over the first week after the peel.

The healing process consists of 4 stages. The first stage occurs over the first 12 hours and consists of facial inflammation. The epidermis becomes leathery and begins to separate from the dermis. The underlying treated dermal layer will become necrotic and being to slough. The applied emollient helps with removing this necrotic skin from the underlying tissues. The second stage is desquamation, which occurs over the next 3 to 7 days (**Figs. 3–9**). This exposes the underlying erythematous dermis. The third stage is reepithelialization, which partially coincides with desquamation and occurs between days 2 through 10 following the peel. Reepithelialization will be demonstrated by the changes in dermal color from bright red to a lighter shade of pink. The final stage is fibroplasia and occurs toward the end of the first week and continues for 12 to 16 weeks after the peel. This final period is when the full benefits of the chemical peel become apparent. During

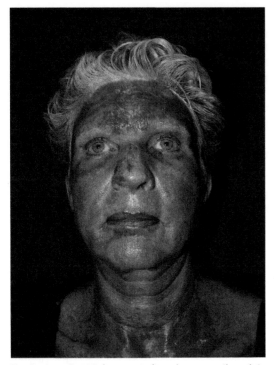

**Fig. 3.** A patient 5 days post phenol-croton oil peel, in the midst of re-epithelialization.

this time, the skin will undergo new collagen formation, reorganization of the collagen, and neoangiogenesis.

For 12 weeks following the peel, the patient is instructed to avoid any direct, prolonged sun exposure. During this period, the skin is vulnerable to UV light exposure and is at risk for resultant hyperpigmentation. The senior author also recommends avoidance of sunscreens for the first 6 weeks. Many chemical sunscreens include the ingredient, para-aminobenzoic acid, which can cause erythema, irritation, and induration of the healing skin. It is also recommended that women avoid birth control pills during this same period, as the increased estrogens can lead to hyperpigmentation.

## COMPLICATIONS

Even with careful technique and appropriate patient selection, it is still possible to encounter a host of potential complications following chemical facial resurfacing. Therefore, it is critical for any practitioner offering chemical peels to be cognizant of any potential complications, as well as the appropriate treatments. This knowledge aids in remedying any undesired effects, and still assists in achieving the desired results.

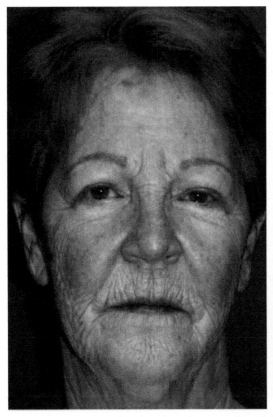
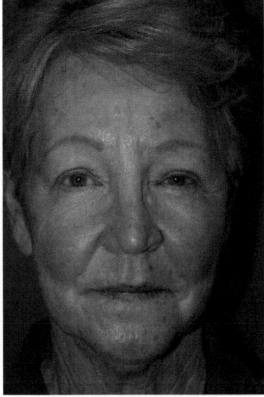

**Fig. 4.** A woman treated with a phenol croton oil peel, improving her fine and course rhytids and skin pigment.

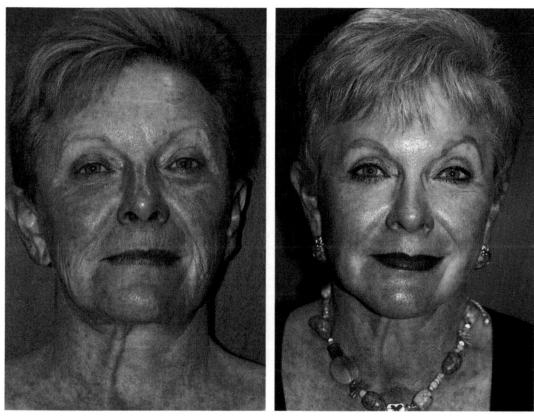

**Fig. 5.** Three months post-phenol croton oil peel, with improvement in skin tone and fine rhytids.

### Cardiac Arrhythmias

The most commonly cautioned and feared intra-operative complication of phenol-croton oil peels is cardiac arrhythmias. Even in patients who have been properly selected and adequately hydrated before their chemical peel, a reversible cardiac arrhythmia can possibly occur. This is especially true in a patient with an undiagnosed

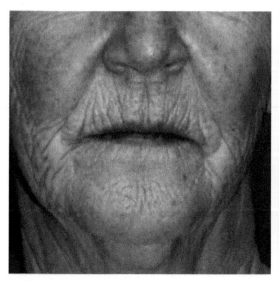

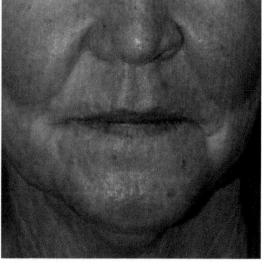

**Fig. 6.** Marked improvement in perioral rhytids following application of a 1.6% Hetter phenol-croton oil peel.

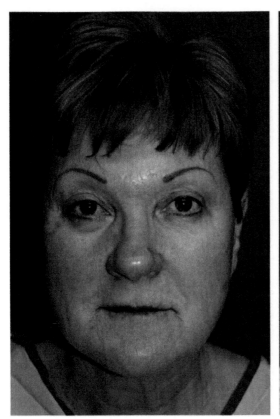 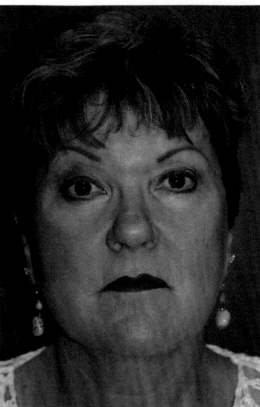

**Fig. 7.** Five months post-peel result with improvements in fine facial rhytids.

heart condition. The common presentation is a supraventricular tachycardia that occurs within 30 minutes of starting the peel, and can evolve into paroxysmal ventricular contractions, paroxysmal atrial tachycardia, ventricular tachycardia, and possibly, atrial fibrillations. The best way to manage any of these listed progressive arrhythmias is to prevent them from occurring in the first place. As soon as a supraventricular tachycardia, or other irregular rhythm, is noted, the peel should be immediately paused and adequate hydration should continue. At this point, the rhythm should eventually return to normal sinus rhythm as the phenol is cleared. Once the rhythm has returned to normal, the phenol peel may proceed carefully with attention to the rhythm monitor. In the rare instance that the rhythm does not naturally return to a normal rhythm, proper medical procedures should be undertaken for that aberrant rhythm.

### Delayed Reepithelialization

A more common complication following a deep chemical peel is prolonged recovery times. Any area of the face that does not fully reepithelialize within 10 days should be considered prolonged. This phenomenon is more common with deeper phenol peels (Baker formula) and TCA peels. It is important to not merely dismiss prolonged healing times as coincidentally, and to rule out the presence of underlying infections or contact irritants. These areas should be checked daily and treated accordingly, or else the risk of scarring can rise precipitously.

### Scarring

If any facial scarring begins to develop, it is most likely to occur in the area of the upper lip or over areas with prominent underlying bone structure such as the mandible. Scarring most commonly is due to an overly deep peel, or from inattentive postoperative care. Again, the risk of scarring is significantly elevated in isotretinoin users. Once the patient has stopped isotretinoin, the practitioner should check to confirm that the patient is clearly producing skin oils. Once developing, the scars can be treated with silicone sheeting coverings and intralesional corticosteroids injections (Kenalog 20 mg/mL) every 2 to

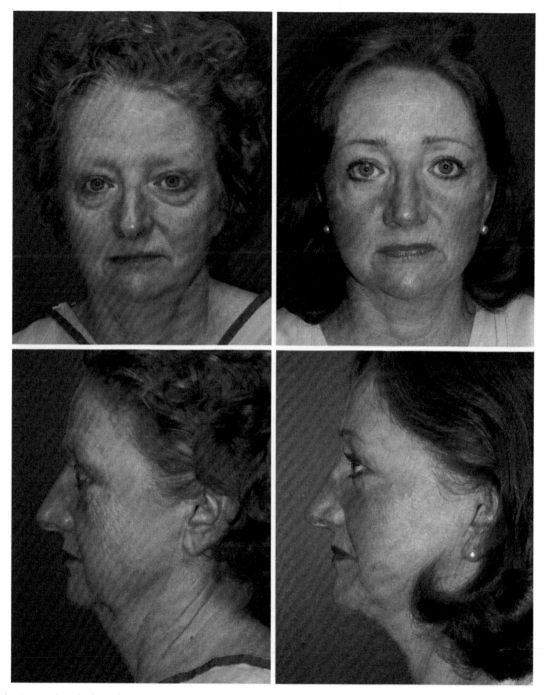

**Fig. 8.** Results of a facelift for a middle-aged woman with excessive submental soft tissue, and moderate jowling.

3 weeks. It is recommended to exercise caution in the injections of steroids, as overinjection can lead to atrophy and skin depressions. As most scars will be erythematous, a flash-lamp pulsed dye laser is helpful over multiple treatments.

### Infections

Bacterial infections can irritate normal wound healing and lead to scar formation. In the case of a patient presenting with signs of cellulitis or infection, an appropriate antibiotic regimen should be immediately started and continued for a 7-day to

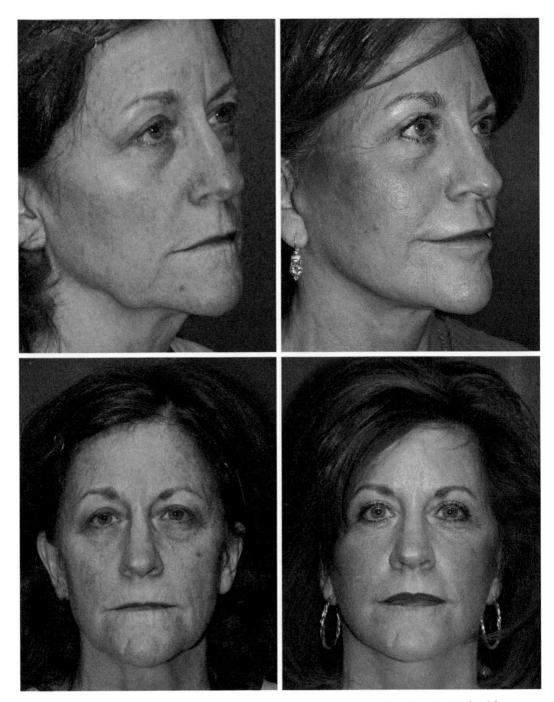

**Fig. 9.** A woman with moderate jowling and neck skin crepiness being treated with an SMAS facelift.

10-day course. Similarly, herpetic viral infections can be problematic for a patient's natural recovery. In the case of a herpetic outbreak despite appropriate prophylactic dosing of antivirals, a course of valacyclovir 1 g 3 times a day for 10 days, should be used.

## Postoperative Erythema

Postoperative erythema after a peel is common in all peel patients and it is not unusual for it to last longer than predicted. In patients with contact dermatitis or sensitive skin, hydrocortisone (2.5%) lotion is commonly prescribed to aid in the resolution of this erythema. As this erythema is eventually subsiding in the weeks following the peel, some patients will develop postinflammatory hyperpigmentation. The typical scenario for this is in a patient with excessive sun exposure following the peel, or with Fitzpatrick III-VI skin types. This can be managed with a combination of 0.05% retinoic acid, 2.5% hydrocortisone cream, and 4% hydroquinone cream.

## *Hypopigmentation*

A more severe complication of chemical peeling is hypopigmentation. This is likely due to phenol's ability to eliminate melanocyte's ability to produce melanin. Hypopigmentation is far more noticeable when single facial subunits are peeled, rather than the whole face. This complication was more common in the past when deeper peels such as the classic Baker formulation were used, along with postoperative occlusive dressing applications. Hypopigmentation is unfortunately irreversible, and all patients who experience some level of this should be advised about the potential need for makeup usage.

## SUMMARY

With the relatively recent arrival of $CO_2$ laser resurfacing and Erbium:YAG laser resurfacing, chemical peeling was disregarded by many as an out-of-date procedure. In addition, phenol-croton oil peels were considered by many to have unpredictable and possibly dangerous results compared with the more recent modalities. Much like the disproven phenol peel dogmas of the twentieth century, these beliefs are far from reality. Phenol-croton oil peeling has withstood the test of time and is still considered the standard against which other facial resurfacing procedures are judged. In addition, the widely expanded knowledge of croton oil, and its various concentrations, has yielded many options for specializing treatment for different facial subunits, skin types, thicknesses, and so on. A strong familiarity with the fundamentals and techniques of chemical peeling can result in predictable and excellent results.

## DISCLOSURE

The authors have nothing to disclose.

## REFERENCES

1. Brody HJ. Complications of chemical peeling. J Dermatol Surg Oncol 1989;15:1010–9.
2. Brody HJ. Complications of chemical resurfacing. Dermatol Clin 2001;19:427–38.
3. Kim IH, Kim HK, Kye YC. Effects of tretinoin pretreatment on TCA chemical peel in guinea pig skin. J Korean Med Sci 1996;11:335–41.
4. Popp C, Kligman AM, Stoudemayer TJ. Pretreatment of photoaged forearm skin with topical tretinoin accelerates healing of full-thickness wounds. Br J Dermatol 1995;132:46–53.
5. Hevia O, Nemeth AJ, Taylor JR. Tretinoin accelerates healing after trichloroacetic acid chemical peel. Arch Dermatol 1986;15:848.
6. Yu RJ, Van Scott EJ. Alpha-hydroxy acids: science and therapeutic use. J Cosmet Dermatol 1994; 1(Suppl 1):12.
7. Van Scott EJ, Yu RJ. Alpha-hydroxy acids: procedures for use in clinical practice. Cutis 1989;43:222.
8. Hayes DK, Berkland ME, Stambough KI. Dermal healing after local skin flaps and chemical peels. Arch Otolaryngol Head Neck Surg 1990;116:794.
9. Brody HJ. Variations and comparisons in medium depth chemical peeling. J Dermatol Surg Oncol 1989;15:953.
10. Dinner MI, Artz JS. Chemical peel: what's in the formula? Plast Reconstr Surg 1994;94:406.
11. Brody HJ. Chemical peeling and resurfacing. St Louis (MO): Mosby; 1997. p. 109–10.
12. Monheit GD. Advances in chemical peeling. Facial Plast Surg Clin North Am 1994;2:5–9.
13. Coleman WP, Futrell JM. The glycolic acid trichloroacetic acid peel. J Dermatol Surg Oncol 1994;20: 76–80.
14. Litton C. Chemical face lifting. Plast Reconstr Surg 1954;13(3):240–5.
15. Hetter GP. An examination of the phenol-crotol oil peel: part III. The plastic surgeon's role. Plast Reconstr Surg 2000;105:752–63.
16. Brown AM, Kaplan LM, Brown ME. Phenol-induced histological skin changes: hazards, technique, and uses. British Journal of Plastic Surgery 1960;13: 158–69.
17. Hetter GP. An examination of the phenol-croton oil peel: part I. Dissecting the formula. Plast Reconstr Surg 2000;105:227–39. discussion 249–251.
18. Johnson JB, Ichinose H, Obagi ZE, et al. Obagi's modified trichloroacetic acid (TCA)-controlled variable-depth peel: a study of clinical signs correlating with histological findings. Ann Plast Surg 1996;36: 225–37.
19. Monheit GD. Medium-depth chemical peels. Dermatol Clin 2001;19:413–25.
20. Szachowicz EH, Wright WK. Delayed healing after full-face chemical peels. Facial Plast Surg 1989;6: 8–13.

# Prescription Skin Care Products and Skin Rejuvenation

William H. Truswell, MD[a,b,c,d],*

## KEYWORDS

- Hyperpigmentation • Aging skin • Retinoids • Hydroquinone • Azelaic acid • Rhytids
- Photodamage • Beauty

## KEY POINTS

- Treatment of aging skin has been pursued by humankind for millennia.
- Intrinsic and extrinsic factors influence the aging process.
- Skin anatomy is key to understanding the aging process.
- Prescriptive treatments are directed at the physiologic processes of aging skin and have clinically proved ability to alter the structure and thereby appearance of the skin.

## INTRODUCTION

The largest organ is not in the human body but on it, the skin. For millennia, humans have been arising in the morning; washing their faces and fixing their hair; dressing in clean, pressed clothes; and, for many, applying makeup and adorning with jewelry. This morning ritual is performed in a way that individuals feel good about how they look and have the expectation that others will react positively to them. For many, part of that morning ritual is cleansing their skin of the face with the best wash and applying toners, conditioners, moisturizers, sun protection, and more, using what are considered the very best products to protect, nourish, and rejuvenate the skin of the face and neck. Skin care products requiring a prescription are classified as drugs.

Drugs are approved by the Food and Drug Administration (FDA) after undergoing an intensive regimen to certify their safety and efficacy. Drugs are substances that affect the structure or function of any bodily part. Cosmetics, on the other hand, are mostly developed by the skin care industry and are not required to undergo such scrutiny. They are under the auspices of the FDA Center for Food Safety and Applied Nutrition, which sets guidelines for their labeling and safety. Cosmetics do not alter the body structures. Cosmeceuticals are over-the-counter products that have some demonstrable effect on the appearance of the skin. Cosmeceuticals are generally available at physicians' offices, neither over the counter nor requiring a prescription. They fall into a gray area between drugs and cosmetics.

## BEAUTY

*Things are beautiful if you love them.*
—Jean Anouilh

That which is beautiful has been analyzed, measured, proportioned, discussed, and debated since the origins of consciousness. Facial plastic surgeons have studied facial appearances. They

---

Disclosure Statement: The author has nothing to disclose.
a Division of Otolaryngology–Head and Neck Surgery, University of Connecticut School of Medicine, Farmington, CT, USA; b American Board of Facial Plastic and Reconstructive Surgery; c American Academy of Facial Plastic and Reconstructive Surgery; d Private Practice, Easthampton, MA, USA
* 123 Union Street, Suite 100, Easthampton, MA 01027.
*E-mail address:* bill.truswell@gmail.com

Facial Plast Surg Clin N Am 28 (2020) 59–65
https://doi.org/10.1016/j.fsc.2019.09.005
1064-7406/20/© 2019 Elsevier Inc. All rights reserved.

have measured, proportioned, and analyzed angles all in the goal to define beauty (**Fig. 1**). That is all to the good, but when we see a beautiful face, we know it instantly without intellectualizing it.

Beauty is ethereal and intangible. Artists strive to create it, architects to build it, composers to assemble it, and facial plastic surgeons to restore it. Beauty exists in nature, large and inspiring as the Grand Canyon in all its permanent glory and tiny and impermanent as a snowflake. When we encounter beauty, we know it before we contemplate it. It is in our hearts before it is in our minds. A heart-shaped face, glowing skin, alluring eyes, and pouting lips—the list of adjectives that are used to describe beauty is legion. But no adjective perfect. There is more to the beauty of a person than that which pleases the eyes. If the demeanor behind the eyes is coarse and unbecoming, the attraction dulls.

Phi, the letter used by the ancient Greeks to describe the golden ratio, which expresses an ideal proportion of 2 aspects of an object, may be that which best describes beauty. Mathematically it is the ratio calculated by dividing a line into 2 parts so that the longer part divided by the smaller part is also equal to the whole length divided by the longer part. In the human face, when the length is approximately 1.5 times longer than the width, the ratio is approximately 1.618, the Golden Ratio. This ratio is found in nature in flower petals, conical shells, in ancient architecture as in the Great Pyramid of Giza, and in art, for example, da Vinci's Last Supper, Vitruvian Man, and Mona Lisa. If you encountered Mona Lisa walking arm in arm with Sophia Loren (or any great modern beauty), which one would catch the eye first?

An interesting contemplation is just how important beauty is in choosing a mate. The physical beauty of a face comes from averaging the features of people of the same age and gender.[1] An averaged face is not unremarkable but rather good looking. It is not common or frequently occurring but familiar. From the Greek words *koinos* (that which is shared) and *philia* (fondness or love), there is *koinophilia*. The term *koinophilia* represents in nature the fact that animals seek mates of average features, because extreme or unnatural features may represent unwanted/unhealthy mutations. Men prefer female faces that are closer to the population average.[2]

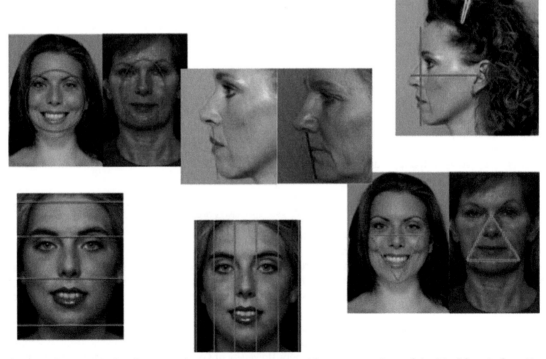

**Fig. 1.** Various proportion lines, angular assessments, and graphic representations of the ideal female face. *Top row, left to right*: (1) The circle of youth, the oval of aging; (2) Full youthful lips forward of the line from columella to mentum. Flattening of lips behind line with age; (3) A vertical line through the horizontal Frankfurt line ideally touches the both glabella and mentum. *Bottom row, left to right*: (4) Equal horizontal thirds of ideal facial proportions; (5) Equal vertical fifths of ideal facial proportions; (6) The inverted triangle of youth, The triangle of age.

In all, I think Jon Anouilh was correct: "Things are beautiful if you love them."

## HISTORICAL PERSPECTIVE

For millennia, women have been applying liquids, potions, powders, abrasives, and cosmetics to the skin of their faces to preserve the beauty of youth and hide the advancement of age by creating an illusion. In ancient Egypt, women would bathe in sour milk. Sour milk is lactic acid, an α-hydroxy acid, which is commonly found in many light chemical peel solutions today. They also used abrasive concoctions containing substances, such as animal oil, alabaster, pumice, and salts; another mixture used is animal oil, lime, and chalk. In Indonesia, women used ground coffee beans as an abrasive. The coffee contains the antioxidant caffeic acid, which tightens collagen fibers and stimulates neocollagenesis. Women in India mixed pumice with urine as a facial scrub. Pumice was the abrasive, and urine contains urea, which is hydrophilic and is used in several cosmetic preparations today.[3] Women all over the world going far back in time experimented with oils, exfoliators, moisturizers, and acids to brighten and rejuvenate their skin.

In the mid-nineteenth century, both medical and lay practitioners began experimenting with other and stronger chemicals as chemoexfoliants and using more aggressive methods of mechanical exfoliation. One of the earliest users of phenol, Dr P.J. Unna, also tried resorcinol, salicylic acid, and trichloroacetic acid.[4] Phenol was also use by Dr Mackee in 1903 for scar treatment. Dr Mackee teamed up with Dr Karp to study the clinical application of phenol, and they published their findings in 1952 in the *British Journal of Dermatology*.[5] These early trials were done mostly in Great Britain and France. Dr la Gasse, in treating World War I injuries from gun powder explosions, placed adhesive tape over the phenol-treated areas. When peeling migrated to America, it was done at first by lay peelers. Formulations of the peeling solutions were held secret, but many used croton oil along with phenol in various ratios.[6,7] The science and technology of modern techniques of skin rejuvenation evolved over many centuries of experimentation with acids, oils, and abrasives. In the last third of the twentieth century, skin rejuvenation techniques changed dramatically with the development of cutaneous lasers.

## ANATOMY OF THE SKIN

The skin is composed of 3 distinct layers: the epidermis, the dermis, and the subdermis (**Fig. 2**). The epidermis is stratified epithelium and has 5

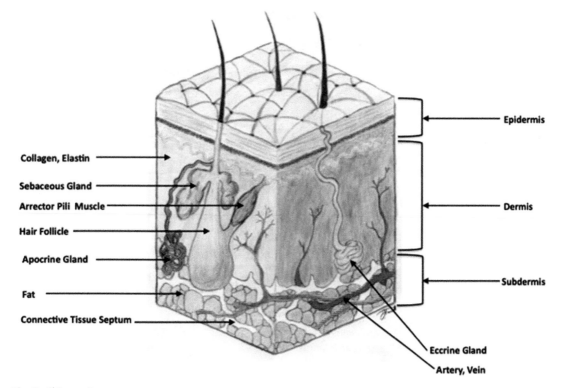

**Fig. 2.** Skin anatomy.

layers. The deepest is the stratum basale, which lies atop the basement membrane and is made up mostly of a single layer of basal cells. Keratinocytes arise here and transition upward through the epidermal layers. Scattered throughout are melanocytes. Epithelial projections, the rete ridges, of the basement membrane interdigitate with dermal papillae anchoring in a sense the epidermis to the dermis. The next layer up is the stratum spinosum followed by the stratum granulosum. The stratum lucidum is a thin layer that transitions between the strati granulosum and corneum. The stratum corneum contains keratinocytes that are without nuclei. The stratum corneum is shed through washing over time. The epidermis is without vascularity. Nutrients diffuse from the dermis to support the viability of the epidermis.

The dermis consists of 2 layers. The papillary dermis is more superficial and contains elastic fibers, loose collagen fibers, reticular fibers, capillaries, and fibroblasts. The thicker, deeper reticular dermis is primarily made up of collagen. Elastin herein lends resilience and elasticity to the skin. Pilosebaceous apparatuses originate in the reticular dermis. These consist of sebaceous, eccrine, and apocrine glands, and hair follicles. The bulb of the hair follicle arising in the reticular dermis extends downward into the subdermis. The hair shaft pushes through all 3 skin layers to rise above the surface of the epidermis. The sebaceous and apocrine glands empty into the follicle. The eccrine glands empty directly onto the surface of the epidermis. The subdermis is a fatty layer that offers insulation to the deeper tissues.[8,9]

## HOW THE SKIN AGES

The eternal question may be: How does the glow of youth, the opalescent, soft, without flaw skin of youth become the thin, dry, brittle, patina painted skin old age? As time goes by, both intrinsic and extrinsic factors influence the onset, rate, and degree of the aging process. The human face ages in 3 ways. The skin shows signs of aging first, followed by tissue descent, and eventually loss of volume.

The glow of youth is due in large part to the fact that the stratum corneum is far less adherent in the first 3 to 4 decades of life. From childhood to the mid to late 30s, when the face is washed, the layer is easily shed. Toward the end of the fourth decade of life, this layer becomes more adherent. As the stratum corneum thickens, the skin becomes duller and flatter. The pores enlarge and are visible. Fine rhytids appear. Lentigines, keratoses, and telangiectasias become apparent. Like all organs, genetic factors take hold over time and effect cellular behavior. The rate of turnover of skin cell slows

and the population of senescent cells multiplies. The time for the keratinocytes in the stratum basale to evolve into the corneocytes of the stratum corneum lengthens, and the ability to re-epithelize is hampered. This is demonstrated by the intolerance of senescent skin to repeated adhesive removal. The aging of the stratum corneum also weakens the epidermal barrier making the skin more permeable to irritants and increasing the risk of contact dermatitis. The rete ridges at the dermal/epidermal junction flatten and shearing injuries occur more commonly. Pigmentary irregularities and loss of hair color occur as the number of melanocytes declines. The sensations of touch and pressure are diminished as the population of Meissner and pacinian corpuscles declines.[10]

Extrinsic factors that contribute and hasten the aging process of the skin include sun exposure and smoking but also chronic illness in particular diabetes, excessive weight loss, and poor nutrition. Foremost among the extrinsic factors contributing to the aging process is sun exposure. Photodamage due to sun exposure and tanning beds is attributable to 80% of the signs of aging skin.[11] Decades of sun exposure contribute to the disorganization of collagen fibers and random thickening of elastin fibers. The skin thickness becomes irregular, thinning in areas and thicker in others. The epidermal adnexa, the apocrine, eccrine, and sebaceous glands decrease in numbers. The skin becomes weathered, dry, brittle, and flakey (**Fig. 3**). As collagen fibers

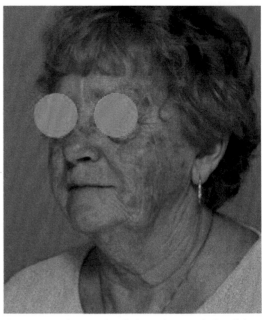

**Fig. 3.** Typical example of photodamaged, dry, flakey, parchment-like skin.

disappear, the dermis thins irregularly and the epidermis drapes over the ridges resulting in fine rhytids. The solar elastosis causes random elastin fiber thickening and stacking of fibers. This causes ridges to form and heavy rhytids become apparent.[8] **Fig. 4** illustrates photographs of a woman in the eighth decade of life. She lived her whole life on a farm and never used sun protection or skin care. The picture on the left shows a parchment-like complexion, fine to coarse rhytides, several keratoses and lentigines, and irregular pigmentation. The picture on the right is a computer-generated simulation of a Wood lamp view, bringing the damaged landscape of the skin of her face into dramatic relief. **Fig. 5** is the artists rendition of senescent skin depicting thinning of the layers, flattening of the rete ridges, loss of adnexa, diminution of vascularity, and surface discolorations and irregularities (see **Fig. 5**).

## PRESCRIPTION SKIN CARE PRODUCTS

Federal Food, Drug, and Cosmetic Act cosmetics are "articles to be rubbed, poured, sprinkled, sprayed on, introduced into or otherwise applied to the body for cleansing, beautifying, promoting attractiveness or altering the appearance." Drugs are defined as "articles intended for use in the diagnosis, cure, mitigation, treatment, or prevention of disease" and "articles intended to affect the structure or any function of the body of man or other animals."[11] The term, *cosmeceutical*, was coined in 1984 by Albert Kligman, MD, PhD, to describe products that had therapeutic benefits for the skin beyond that which cosmetics could offer. They can change the biologic function of the skin. They have true clinical abilities to rejuvenate and repair photodamaged skin. Typically, they can be sold in a physician's office but not in stores. As such, they fall in that space between cosmetics and drugs.[12]

### Hydroquinone

Hydroquinone, a phenolic compound (1,4 dihydroxybenzene), is commonly used in the United States in the treatment of melasma and postinflammatory hyperpigmentation (PIH). It is available over the counter in 2% solutions and in 4% to 10% solutions by prescription. It works by blocking the

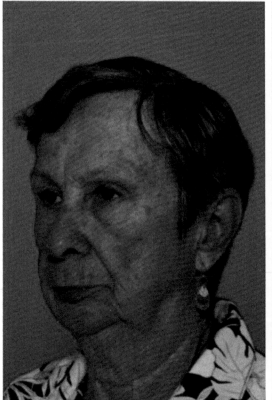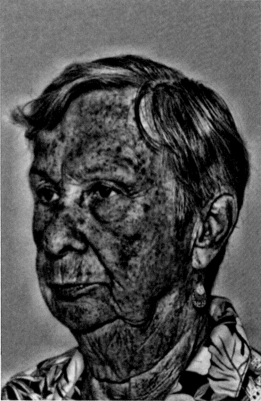

**Fig, 4.** (*Left*) A 75-year-old woman with lifelong unprotected sun exposure with excessive photodamage. (*Right*) A computer-generated simulation of a Wood lamp view of the same face bringing the signs aging and photo-damaged skin into relief.

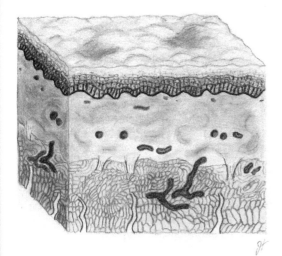

**Fig. 5.** Senescent skin with flattening of the rete ridges, loss of adnexa, diminution of vascularity, and surface discolorations and irregularities.

conversion of dihydroxyphenylalanine to tyrosinase, thus stopping the synthesis of melanin. It is thought to inhibit the synthesis of DNA and RNA. It also may be selectively cytotoxic to melanocytes and initiate degradation of melanosomes by autooxidation and phenol oxidases. That process prevents the production of melanin and inhibits the transfer of melanin to the keratinocytes.[13]

Hydroquinone, 4%, is the standard treatment of both melasma and PIH. It has been administered for more than 50 years. It has been banned over the past 10 years or so years, however, in the European Union, Japan, and Australia. There is the possible risk of development of cancer in mice and liver or nerve damage. Ochronosis is another real but rare risk that has been reported in blacks in South Africa. The FDA has explored banning over-the-counter sale of hydroquinone but not yet acted. Hydroquinone gradually reduces hyperpigmentation. Its clinical efficacy becomes apparent at 20 weeks. At 6 months, this efficacy levels off. It is applied to the entire face twice daily (spot treatment produces a bull's-eye effect).[13,14]

For more severe or persistent hyperpigmentation, combination therapy for hydroquinone with retinoids or mequinol may be appropriate. Pathak and colleagues[15] found that 0.1% tretinoin combined with 2% hydroquinone to be used at night was the most effective. When a satisfactory outcome is still not achieved, triple therapy is started adding a topical steroid. An effective product for both PIH and melasma contains 4% hydroquinone, 0.05% tretinoin, and 0.01% fluocinolone (commercially Tri-Luma Cream, Galderma, Fort Worth, Texas) is used for 2 months.

When topical steroid cream is used longer than 8 weeks, telangiectasias and steroid induced acne can occur. After 8 weeks, patients can hydroquinone and tretinoin. If no recurrence is apparent at 12 months, tretinoin cream can be used nightly.[13]

### Tretinoin (Retinoic Acid)

Of the 3 primary vitamin A derivatives, retinol is an alcohol, retinal is an aldehyde, and tretinoin is retinoic acid. Retinol is available over the counter for treatment of photodamaged and aging skin. Retinal is a less irritating form and is important for vision. Tretinoin is the prescriptive form for dermatologic use to improve aging skin and lessen the effects of solar damage. Tretinoin reverses the effects of photodamage and aging in half the time as retinol. Aging skin is rough, shows dyschromia, and exhibits fine to course rhytids. UV light hastens development of all of these characteristics of aging of skin.[16]

At least a dozen double-blind studies have attested to the clinical efficacy of topical retinoids. Tretinoin is absorbed through the skin and becomes bound to retinoic acid receptors in the nuclei and moderate gene expression. Collagen production is increased by these processes. Matrix metalloproteinase enzymes in the skin are responsible for collagen degradation and slowing collagen synthesis. These enzymes are increased by UV light accelerating the aging effects. Retinoids block these enzymes thus providing a second pathway to collagen production. Tretinoin has positive effects on both the epidermis and epidermis. The appearance and tactile feel of the skin improve with thinning of the epidermis, lessening of corneocyte adhesion, and decreasing melanocyte production. In the dermis there is an increase in the amount of collagen, decrease in the amount of collagenase, and increase of the glycosaminoglycans. The skin color lightens and fine and coarse rhytids decrease.[12,16] Side effects include stinging, burning, redness and peeling. These effects dissipate over time of use. The application can be lessened to every other day or even halted to be resumed when the symptoms improve. It is important to continue good skin. Tretinoin should be applied at night time, sun block is imperative daily long with good moisturizers.

### Mequinol

Mequinol is 4-hydroxyanisole and is approved for prescriptive use in the United States. It is less irritating then hydroquinone and may be substituted for it if hydroquinone has proved too irritating for a patient. It is an inhibitor of tyrosinase, thus blocking the formation of melanin. It is available in a 2% solution. It often is compounded with tretinoin 0.01%, which enhances its penetration. It can be used in most skin types.[13] In 2004, Piacquadio[17] published a study comparing 2% mequinol/0.01% tretinoin solution with 4% hydroquinone. He concluded both were equally effective.

## Arbutin/Deoxyarbutin

Arbutin is the natural compound from blueberry, cranberry, and bearberry leaves. Arbutin is a synthetically produced form. It acts by the inhibition of tyrosinase and inhibiting the maturation of melanosome. Deoxyarbutin has higher tyrosinase inhibition. There are few human trials for PIH reported but some consider it the most effective skin lightning agent. Its effect is reversible when discontinued.[13,18]

## Azelaic Acid

Azelaic acid, 1.7-heptane dicarboxylic acid, is available in 2 prescriptive strengths, 15% and 20%. The 15% solution is used for mild to moderate papulopustular acne rosacea. The 20% preparation is prescribed for acne vulgaris, melasma, and PIH. It works as a skin lightning agent by inhibiting tyrosinase probably by inhibiting mitochondrial oxidoreductase activity.[13]

## Eflornithine Hydrochloride

Eflornithine hydrochloride (commercially Vaniqa Cream, SkinMedica, Irvine, California) is an FDA-approved prescriptive product that decreases the growth of unwanted facial hair in women by inhibiting ornithine decarboxylase. It does not eliminate hair growth. It must be applied twice daily. Results become apparent after a considerable period of time.[19]

## REFERENCES

1. Halberstadt J, Pecher D, Zeelenberg R, et al. Two faces of attractiveness: making beauty in averageness appear and reverse. Psychol Sci 2013;24(11): 2343–6.
2. Munoz-Reyes JA, Iglesias-Julios M, Pita M, et al. Facial features: what women perceive as attractive and what men consider attractive. PLoS One 2015; 10(7):e0132979.
3. King BJ. The history and evolution of skin resurfacing. In: Truswell WH, editor. Lasers and light, peels and abrasions – applications and techniques. New York: Thieme Medical Publishers; 2016. p. 1–7.
4. Brody HJ. History of chemical peels. In: Brody HJ, editor. Chemical peeling. St Louis (MO): Mosby-Year Book, Inc.; 1992. p. 1–5.
5. Mackee GM, Karp FL. The treatment of post acne scars with phenol. Br J Dermatol 1952;64:456–9.
6. Hetter GP. An examination of the phenol-croton oil peel: part I. dissecting the formula. Plast Reconstr Surg 2000;105(1):227–39.
7. Hetter GP. An examination of the phenol-croton oil peel: part II. the lay peelers and their croton oil formulas. Plast Reconstr Surg 2000;105(1): 240–8.
8. Truswell WH, Fox AJ. Sataloff's comprehensive textbook of otolaryngology head & neck surgery. In: Sataloff RT, editor. Facial plastic and reconstructive surgery, vol. 3. New Delhi (India): Jaypee Brothers Medical Publishers Ltd; 2016. p. 365–84.
9. Grobman AB, Harirchian S, Grunebaum LD. Anatomy, physiology, and pathology of the skin. In: Truswell WH, editor. Lasers and light, peels and abrasions – applications and techniques. New York: Thieme Medical Publishers; 2016. p. 8–13.
10. Uitto J. Understanding premature skin aging. N Engl J Med 1997;337:1463.
11. Available at: https://www.fda.gov/Cosmetics/GuidanceRegulation/LawsRegulations/ucm074201.htm. Accessed November 13, 1997.
12. Hessler JL. Anti-aging products and cosmeceuticals. In: Truswell WH, editor. Lasers and light, peels and abrasions – applications and techniques. New York: Thieme Medical Publishers; 2016. p. 273–6.
13. Rossi AM, Perez MI. Treatment of hyperpigmentation. Facial Plast Surg Clin North Am 2011;19: 313–24.
14. Draelos Z. Hydroquinone: optimizing therapeutic outcomes in the clinical setting of melanin-related hyperpigmentation. Today's Therapeutic Trends 2001;19:191–203.
15. Pathak MA, Fitzpatrick TB, Kraus EW. Usefulness of retinoic acid in the treatment of melasma. J Am Acad Dermatol 1986;15:894–9.
16. Clark A, Hessler JL. Skin care. Facial Plast Surg Clin North Am 2015;23:285–95.
17. Piacquadio D. Mequinol 2%/tretinoin 0.01% solution monotherapy and combination treatment of solar lentigines and postinflammatory hyperpigmentation. J Am Acad Dermatol 2004;52(Suppl):P175.
18. Visscher MO, Pan BS, Kitzmiller J. Photodamage treatments and topicals for facial skin. Facial Plast Surg Clin North Am 2013;21:61–75.
19. Hovenic W, DeSpain J. Laser hair reduction and removal. Facial Plast Surg Clin North Am 2011;19: 325–33.

# Plasma Energy Skin Rejuvenation

J. David Holcomb, MD

## KEYWORDS

- Cold atmospheric plasma • Nitrogen plasma skin regeneration • Helium plasma skin regeneration
- Radiofrequency energy • Radiofrequency bridge

## KEY POINTS

- Helium plasma energy is delivered to the tissue in a bimodal fashion via thermal convection/conduction and an ionized helium radiofrequency bridge.
- Animal studies demonstrate greater skin tissue contraction for helium plasma versus nitrogen plasma, likely resulting from greater energy density for helium plasma.
- Clinical use of helium plasma for skin rejuvenation demonstrates significant skin tightening and rhytid reduction, high patient satisfaction, and manageable side effects/complications.
- Helium plasma skin regeneration may be safely performed concurrently with various surgical facial rejuvenation procedures but should be staged ideally before injectable soft tissue filler injections.
- Indications, contraindications, efficacy, and side effects/complications for helium plasma energy skin rejuvenation are similar to deep laser skin resurfacing treatments except that treatment must be avoided in patients with implanted electrical devices.

 Video content accompanies this article at http://www.facialplastic.theclinics.com.

## INTRODUCTION

A new form of plasma energy skin rejuvenation is emerging as a promising tool in doctors' skin resurfacing armamentariums. Helium plasma skin regeneration (PSR) uses radiofrequency (RF) energy to "activate" helium gas to deliver thermal energy to the skin in a bimodal fashion with direct heating of the skin's surface by the flow of hot (ionized and nonionized) helium gas as well as Joule (resistive) heating of dermal tissue below the surface by the flow of electrical current that propagates from the hand-piece tip (cathode) to the target tissue (anode) through the flow of ionized helium. The flow of RF energy to the tissue requires electrical coupling between the treatment tip and the skin, and this occurs passively only for a short distance from the skin's surface (eg, <10 mm). Treatment tip distance to the skin's surface within the electrical coupling range is not thought to significantly impact energy density. Targeted areas of the skin are treated completely, that is, full field treatment. Although energy deposition is full field, the flow of energy to the skin's surface is dependent on continuously changing skin tissue impedance (immediately increases at treated areas) that also limits depth of effect.[1]

The predicate Nitrogen PSR device also uses RF energy to heat a flow of nitrogen gas in the treatment tip. The flowing nitrogen gas is partially ionized and then pulsed onto the skin's surface wherein convective heating of the tissue surface then results in conductive heat transfer into the dermis. Joule tissue heating does not occur with nitrogen PSR treatment. Treatment tip to skin offsets distance directly and predictably impacts

Disclosure: Dr J. David Holcomb is a consultant for Apyx Medical Corporation.
Holcomb – Kreithen Plastic Surgery and MedSpa, 1 South School Avenue, Suite 800, Sarasota, FL 34237, USA
E-mail address: drholcomb@sarasota-med.com

Facial Plast Surg Clin N Am 28 (2020) 67–74
https://doi.org/10.1016/j.fsc.2019.09.006

heat transfer and energy density because a greater offset distance allows more time for the heated nitrogen gas/plasma to cool before impacting the skin's surface. To take advantage of this phenomenon, a very low energy treatment protocol was developed that incorporates a treatment tip attachment that significantly increases offset distance.[2] Although the entire surface of the skin is treated, the Guassian nature of the energy pulse results in uneven energy deposition with a central hotspot within each pulse.

Nitrogen PSR treatment has demonstrated excellent clinical efficacy for treatment of photodamage[2–8] and modest clinical efficacy for scarring (acne[9] and traumatic[10]) and wrinkle reduction.[3–6,8,11] Safety of nitrogen PSR treatment and concurrent surgical procedures (eg, brow lift, cheek augmentation, and facelift surgery, including lower-energy, single-pass treatment of undermined skin) has also been demonstrated.[4] Nitrogen PSR treatment is nonablative at the time of treatment with immediate desiccation of the upper layers of skin that remain intact during initial healing and subsequently slough revealing newly regenerated skin with improved dermal architecture.[12] Although initial healing with reepithelialization typically occurs within 7 to 10 days, instances of delayed healing have been experienced with higher energy levels (eg, 3.0–4.0 J) with both single-pass (PSR2) and double-pass (PSR3) treatment over peripheral areas of the face (upper forehead, temples, posterior cheeks, jawline). Along with efficacy and safety, additional factors that have helped to solidify acceptance of nitrogen PSR technology include the lack of an open wound during optimal healing, suitable protocol diversity for various skin conditions and skin types (eg, Fitzpatrick I, II, III, IV), and a relative paucity of significant treatment complications.

Animal studies comparing skin tissue effects of the novel helium PSR technology with the predicate nitrogen PSR device demonstrated similarity of histologic findings for the plasmas but reduced depth of thermal effect, reduced depth of reparative tissue healing, and greater skin tissue contraction immediately after and 30 days after treatment of the helium plasma technology.[13] Reduced depth of effect for the novel helium PSR technology may be explained by lateral spread of helium plasma RF energy (impedance of treated tissue increases resulting in lateral spread of helium plasma RF energy to adjacent untreated, lower-impedance tissue) and the relatively low current RF energy needed to ionize helium gas (current dispersed quickly and therefore unable to penetrate deep into the tissue). The enhanced skin tissue contraction (plasma beam coagulation) observed by the novel helium PSR technology may be explained by increased energy density (bimodal energy deposition, smaller treatment tip, relatively shallow depth of thermal effect) and also points to suitability for use in skin resurfacing procedures.

### Helium Plasma Skin Regeneration: About the Device

The helium gas plasma soft tissue coagulation device (Renuvion®; Apyx Medical, Clearwater, FL, USA; **Fig. 1**) is cleared by the Food and Drug Administration (FDA) for soft tissue ablation, coagulation, and cutting. Adjustable treatment variables include power (percent), helium gas flow rate (L/min), and pulsing (both on duration and off duration in milliseconds) (**Fig. 2**). A single-use, disposable 44-mm treatment hand piece is available for use in skin resurfacing (**Fig. 3**). The plasma beam may be activated by a button on the hand piece or a foot pedal. The treatment tip must be placed within the electrical coupling range that extends only a short distance from the skin's surface for plasma beam coagulation to occur. As excited electrons fall back to their ground states, photons are released that result in visibility of the plasma beam (violet white; **Fig. 4**), a phenomenon known as the Lewis-Rayleigh afterglow that also occurs with the nitrogen PSR device but at a different wavelength and color (yellow visible light).

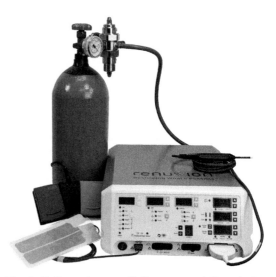

Fig. 1. Helium plasma soft tissue coagulation device with attached helium gas tank, 44-mm long hand piece (treatment tip) for energy delivery, foot pedal for helium plasma beam activation, and grounding pad. (*Courtesy of* Apyx Medical Corporation, Clearwater, FL, USA; with permission.)

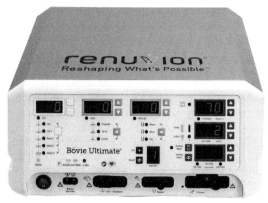

**Fig. 2.** Control (*front*) panel of helium plasma soft tissue coagulation device. The helium plasma (Renuvion®) controls are on the right side and outlined in purple: J-PLASMA Power % (*top*), GAS FLOW L/min (*middle*), PULSING ON TIME and OFF TIME (*bottom*). (*Courtesy of* Apyx Medical Corporation, Clearwater, FL, USA; with permission.)

## HELIUM PLASMA SKIN REGENERATION: TREATMENT CONCEPTS
### Indications and Contraindications

The helium plasma device has received FDA 510(k) clearance and a general indication for cutting, coagulation, and ablation of soft tissue during

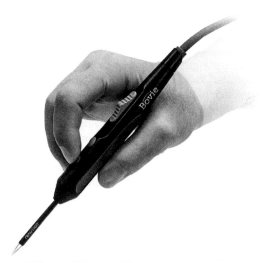

**Fig. 3.** Helium plasma hand piece with 44-mm long treatment tip. Note that this dual-purpose hand piece allows for both helium plasma coagulation (blade retracted, purple activator button) and soft tissue cutting (blade extended, purple and blue activator buttons with blue providing standard monopolar coagulation with helium – CoolCoag™). A single-purpose dermal resurfacing hand piece with the same dimensions but with only a recessed electrode in the treatment tip (no extendable blade) is awaiting regulatory approval. (*Courtesy of* Apyx Medical Corporation, Clearwater, FL, USA; with permission.)

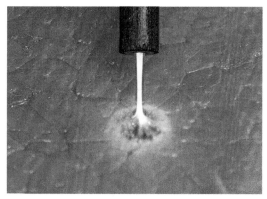

**Fig. 4.** View of helium plasma violet white "beam" coagulating soft tissue (filet mignon). (*Courtesy of* Apyx Medical Corporation, Clearwater, FL; with permission.)

open and laparoscopic surgical procedures. At the time of this writing, use of the device for the indication of dermal resurfacing is exclusively off-label. The author's approach to off-label use of the helium PSR device is similar to his approach for deep skin resurfacing with the dual mode erbium-YAG laser. His algorithm for deep skin resurfacing includes appropriate skin type and skin condition, absence of absolute (and ideally relative) contraindications, and patient acceptance of downtime and procedure-specific risks. The author prefers to treat Fitzpatrick skin types I, II, and III but will occasionally treat Fitzpatrick skin type IV, although less aggressively. The author currently restricts this newer treatment to those patients with significant skin laxity, rhytidosis, and photoaging. He delays treating patients who have been on Accutane in the past year. For deep resurfacing treatments, patients must be willing to undergo up to 2 weeks of downtime for reepithelialization and accept risks of deep skin resurfacing, including delayed healing, scarring, prolonged erythema, and dyschromia (hyperpigmentation, hypopigmentation).

Absolute contraindications for treatment include those for laser skin resurfacing (eg, active skin infection, isotretinoin use in past 12 months, immunosuppression, melasma, suspicious skin lesion or skin cancer in treatment area, insufficient downtime available for recovery, unrealistic expectations regarding treatment benefits and outcomes)[14] but also notably include patients who are ineligible for treatments involving monopolar RF energy (eg, cardiac pacemaker). Relative contraindications for treatment also include those for laser skin resurfacing (collagen vascular disease, abnormal scarring, prior radiation therapy or deep burn in treatment area, diffuse hyperpigmentation, Koebnerizing skin conditions, inflammatory condition of the skin, severe skin sensitivity, severe lower eyelid laxity, and prior lower eyelid surgery).[14]

### Pretreatment Considerations

Full-face deep helium PSR treatment may be completed with oral/intramuscular medications, regional nerve blocks, and tumescent local anesthesia. As with perioral laser skin resurfacing,[15] patients undergoing helium PSR treatment in the perioral area undergo prophylaxis against herpes virus infection with an appropriate antiviral therapy. Full-face helium PSR treatment often results in significant initial posttreatment edema, especially in the periorbital area; therefore, patients are given a 6-day oral prednisolone miniburst and taper starting with 24-mg initial dose to mitigate and reduce related discomfort. Although controversial,[16] most patients, especially those also undergoing concurrent surgical procedures, are also prescribed a 1-week course of prophylactic oral antibiotic. Although pretreatment topical skin therapy with alpha-hydroxy acids, tretinoin, and hydroquinone may have little impact on the incidence of postinflammatory hyperpigmentation,[17] pretreatment topical skin therapy with extracellular matrix (ECM) modulators may be beneficial for optimizing healing and outcomes with respect to ECM remodeling.[18]

### Treatment: Skin Preparation

Isolated helium PSR treatment may be performed in a well-ventilated room with a comfortable, adjustable treatment chair/table and adequate lighting. Certainly, helium PSR treatment may also be performed concurrently with various surgical procedures. In either case, the skin should be prepared gently with an appropriate antimicrobial and then wiped clean with sterile saline. The skin surface should be dry at the time of treatment and TOPICAL ANESTHESIA SHOULD NOT BE USED because it will substantially impact skin tissue impedance and unpredictably affect energy delivery. Because topical anesthesia is not used, procedure efficiency is excellent for the treating facility.

### Treatment: Anesthesia and Safety Considerations

Full-face helium PSR treatment may be comfortably and safely performed with oral and/or intramuscular medications (eg, anxiolytic/sedative and/or narcotic pain medication), regional (trigeminal) nerve and labial blocks, and tumescent anesthesia diffusely infiltrated subcutaneously (not intradermal) throughout the treatment areas. Video 1 briefly demonstrates infiltration of tumescent anesthesia in the perioral area. For patients who will be awake during the procedure, initial regional, labial, and peripheral "ring" blocks may be performed with 1% lidocaine containing 1:100,000 epinephrine with sodium bicarbonate added up to 1 part in 10. Tumescent solution is easily prepared by mixing 1% lidocaine containing 1:100,000 epinephrine, 0.5% Marcaine (plain), and sterile saline solution to give final concentrations of 0.25% lidocaine, 0.125% Marcaine, and 1:400,000 epinephrine. Tumescent solution is infiltrated using a 10-cc syringe with attached single-use 23-gauge GEMS Tulip SuperLuerLokinjector. Patient comfort may be enhanced by serially infiltrating and immediately treating each area of the face, for example, forehead, then nose and periorbital, then right cheek, followed by left cheek, and finally the perioral area. Typical tumescent infiltration volume for the face is 50 cc to 75 cc. For patients undergoing intravenous sedation with an oral airway or nasal trumpet, supplemental oxygen should be turned off and oxygen tubing removed during treatment. If a laryngeal mask airway or endotracheal tube is in place, oxygen flow rate should be reduced and the tube should be wrapped with a wet towel during treatment.

### Treatment: Device Settings and Energy Delivery

Device settings and energy delivery should be customized for each patient's skin type, skin condition, and treatment goals. Although available power (percent) ranges from 5% to 100%, typical settings range from 20% to 40%. Adjusting the power level up or down will increase or decrease the depth of effect, respectively. The default helium gas flow rate is set to 4.0 L per minute. Increasing or decreasing the helium gas flow rate does not appear to correlate with depth of effect. Increasing the helium gas flow rate above the default rate may slightly lengthen the RF bridge tissue interface (electrical coupling) distance beyond 5 mm. The default "continuous mode" for energy deposition is a proprietary RF waveform. The proprietary RF waveform may be adjusted by using a pulsing mode wherein the user has the ability to control both the duration of the pulse *on time* and pulse *off time* in milliseconds with a range for each from 20 milliseconds to 980 milliseconds. Using the same relatively short values for both pulse *on time* and pulse *off time* (eg, 20 milliseconds on, 20 milliseconds off) effectively reduces energy density and may improve endpoint reliability and safety. As helium PSR is a nascent technology, no consensus agreement regarding optimal treatment settings yet exists. Video 2 briefly demonstrates adjustment of helium plasma device settings. The recommended method of helium plasma energy deposition onto the skin's surface involves unidirectional linear adjacent passes with no overlap.

## Treatment: Endpoint

Treatment endpoint depends on skin condition, skin type, and treatment goals. Treatment with the predicate device (nitrogen PSR) involved single- or double-pass treatment, wherein the outer layers of skin were desiccated but remained intact during initial healing. Helium PSR single-pass treatment is similar in concept with desiccation of the outer skin layers that remain intact during the initial healing phase. Video 3 demonstrates energy delivery and skin tissue changes with first-pass helium PSR treatment. Because the desiccated skin layers slough over 4 to 10 or more days following treatment, the newly regenerated skin becomes visible. For greater skin tightening and greater improvement of rhytidosis, a second pass may be performed. IT IS VERY IMPORTANT HOWEVER THAT THE DESICCATED OUTER SKIN LAYERS ARE WIPED AWAY WITH MOIST GAUZE BEFORE PERFORMING A SECOND PASS. Failure to remove the desiccated outer skin tissue layers will result in very unpredictable energy delivery owing to significant impedance changes in the desiccated skin tissue (see later discussion, Management of Complications).

After wiping away the desiccated outer skin tissue layers, second-pass helium PSR treatment results in immediately visible skin tightening and a chamois color of the skin that indicates skin desiccation from energy penetration deep into the papillary or upper reticular dermis (as previously documented for the $CO_2$ laser[19]). Because performance of a second pass requires removal of the already treated, desiccated, and still intact superficial tissue (the "biologic dressing"), the appearance of the skin immediately after the second-pass treatment is similar to that of a deep laser skin resurfacing treatment. It is common practice to treat some areas of the face with a single pass, leaving the biologic dressing in place while performing a second pass over areas that require deeper treatment. Video 4 demonstrates wiping away of the desiccated skin tissue after the initial pass and then performance of a second pass in the perioral area. **Figs. 5–8** demonstrate substantial tissue remodeling with significant skin tightening and reduction of rhytidosis.

## Helium Plasma Skin Regeneration as a Concurrent Treatment

Helium PSR may be performed concurrently with facial surgery, including brow lift, transconjunctival lower blepharoplasty, upper blepharoplasty, facelift, and cheek or chin augmentation procedures. Coronal, hairline approach, endoscopic and direct brow lift procedures may be performed immediately preceding helium PSR treatment of the forehead with mild to modest settings (eg, single pass, up to 40% power with pulsing; eg, 20 milliseconds *on time* and 20 milliseconds *off time*). Facelift procedures may also be performed immediately preceding helium PSR treatment. Similar to concurrent nitrogen PSR[4] or laser skin resurfacing[20] procedures, the energy density should be limited (eg, single pass, 20% power with pulsing; eg, 20 milliseconds *on time* and 20 milliseconds *off time*) over thinner, noncomposite flaps, especially in smokers or if any concern about potential impact on flap viability. To ensure flap viability, lower eyelid skin should not be treated with helium PSR concurrently with transcutaneous lower eyelid surgery. Facial injectable procedures should be staged (ideally after) helium PSR treatment to avoid dilution issues for deep dermal

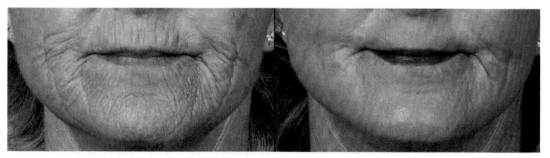

**Fig. 5.** Before (*left*) and after (*right*) photographs: 5 months following facelift and perioral helium PSR at 60% power, 4 L/min gas flow, pulsing (20 milliseconds on, 20 milliseconds off), 2 passes with wiping of desiccated soft tissue between passes. Note marked improvement of vertical lip lines and perioral rhytids.

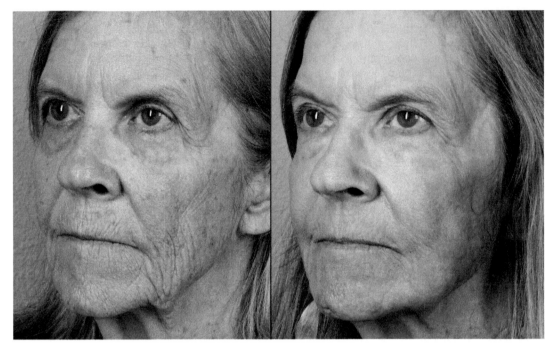

**Fig. 6.** Before (*left*) and after (*right*) photographs: 6 months following full-face helium PSR at 30% power, 4 L/min gas flow, pulsing (20 milliseconds on, 20 milliseconds off), single pass except 2 passes in perioral area with wiping of desiccated soft tissue between passes. Note marked improvement of vertical lip lines and facial rhytids along with reversal of photodamage and significant skin tightening along jaw line and periorbital areas.

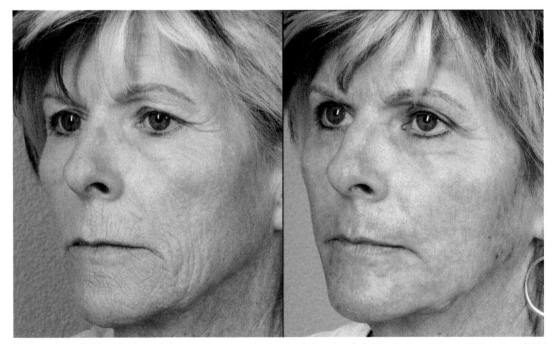

**Fig. 7.** Before (*left*) and after (*right*) photographs: 4 months following full-face helium PSR at 40% power (60% power in perioral area), 4 L/min gas flow, pulsing (20 milliseconds on, 20 milliseconds off), single pass except two passes in perioral area with wiping of desiccated soft tissue between passes. Note marked improvement of vertical lip lines and facial rhytids along with reversal of photodamage and significant skin tightening along jaw line and periorbital areas (surgical upper eyelid blepharoplasty was NOT performed). Note several telangiectasias over the left posterior cheek and noncoalescent erythema in the perioral area.

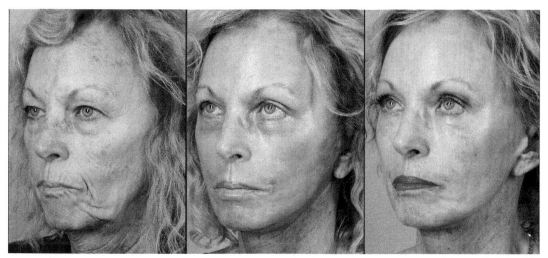

**Fig. 8.** Before (*left*), interim (*center*), and after (*right*) photographs: 6 months following face and neck lift with helium PSR over forehead, nose, periorbital, perioral and medial cheek areas (60% power, 4 L/min gas flow), pulsing (20 milliseconds on, 20 milliseconds off), single pass except 2 passes over cutaneous upper and lower lip areas with wiping of desiccated soft tissue between passes. Note marked improvement of vertical lip lines and perioral rhytids along with reversal of photodamage and significant skin tightening in periorbital areas (surgical upper eyelid blepharoplasty was NOT performed). Note several telangiectasias over the left mid cheek and noncoalescent erythema in the treated areas.

injectables and the potential for unpredictable outcomes with more superficial intradermal injections.

### Posttreatment Skin/Wound Care

During the initial healing period, the treated skin must be kept moist with an occlusive balm (eg, petrolatum with microcrystalline wax, triterpenes, bisabolol, Physalis Angulata extract). The desiccated outer skin layers will slough in approximately 4 to 10 days as the newly regenerated skin appears. Focal areas of slower healing may be apparent beyond 10 days; these areas may be spot treated with an occlusive balm, with silver sulfadiazine or with a biologic membrane to promote more rapid tissue regeneration (eg, Cytal Wound Matrix). After reepithelialization, the occlusive balm is discontinued and both a light moisturizer and ECM modulators are started. Significant sun exposure and harsh wind conditions should be avoided for 6 or more weeks after healing. Mineral-based camouflage makeup may be started soon after reepithelialization, and nonirritating sunscreen may be applied as soon as 3 to 4 weeks after healing.

### Avoidance and Management of Complications

Complications related to helium PSR treatment include hyperpigmentation, hypopigmentation, prolonged erythema, telangiectasia formation, delayed healing, and scarring (atrophic vs

hypertrophic). Although delayed healing and scarring may be avoided by attempting to maintain a reasonable and homogenous energy density (ie, avoiding overtreatment), redness, hypervascularity, and dyschromias must be managed (expectantly vs proactively). As previously mentioned, if a second pass is planned, then the desiccated debris that remains after the initial pass must be wiped away with wet gauze before the second pass is performed. **Figs. 7** and **8** show scattered telangiectasias and persistent erythema that were treated with a 532-nm potassium titanyl phosphate and long-pulse 1064-nm Nd:YAG lasers.

### SUMMARY

Helium PSR is an effective treatment option to combat aging facial skin. Helium plasma's efficacy may be explained by its bimodal energy deposition, unique delivery system, and high energy density. Although single-pass helium PSR treatment depth of effect at moderate power levels is less than for high energy, double-pass nitrogen PSR in animal models, the ability to wipe away the desiccated outer tissue layers and perform a second pass enable clinical outcomes and patient satisfaction to surpass those of the predicate device and of fractional ablative fractional laser treatments and to closely resemble those of deep laser skin resurfacing. Indications, contraindications, and side effects/complications for helium PSR are similar to deep laser skin resurfacing treatments except that helium plasma treatment must be avoided in patients with implanted electrical devices. Helium PSR may be safely performed concurrently with various surgical facial rejuvenation procedures but should be ideally staged before injectable soft tissue filler injections. As doctors' experience with helium plasma energy skin rejuvenation increases, optimum treatment settings and protocols for various skin types and conditions will gradually emerge. The future of skin resurfacing and rejuvenation very likely includes a violet white afterglow.

## SUPPLEMENTARY DATA

Supplementary data related to this article can be found online at https://doi.org/10.1016/j.fsc.2019.09.006.

## REFERENCES

1. Holcomb JD, Schucker A. Helium plasma skin regeneration: evaluation of skin tissue effects in a porcine model and comparison to nitrogen plasma skin regeneration. Lasers Surg Med 2019. [Epub ahead of print].
2. Bernstein EF. Very low energy plasma skin resurfacing treatments improve photodamage. Lasers Surg Med 2007;39(Suppl 19):17.
3. Foster KW, Moy RL, Fincher FF. Advances in plasma skin regeneration. J Cosmet Dermatol 2008;7(3):169–79.
4. Holcomb JD, Kent KJ, Rousso DE. Nitrogen plasma skin regeneration and aesthetic facial surgery: multicenter evaluation of concurrent treatment. Arch Facial Plast Surg 2009;11(3):184–93.
5. Kilmer S, Semchyshyn N, Shah G, et al. A pilot study on the use of a plasma skin regeneration device (Portrait PSR3) in full facial rejuvenation procedures. Lasers Med Sci 2007;22(2):101–9.
6. Elsaie ML, Kammer JN. Evaluation of plasma skin regeneration technology for cutaneous remodeling. J Cosmet Dermatol 2008;7(4):309–11.
7. Bogle MA, Arndt KA, Dover JS. Evaluation of plasma skin regeneration technology in low-energy full-facial rejuvenation. Arch Dermatol 2007;143(2):168–74.
8. Bentkover SH. Plasma skin resurfacing: personal experience and long-term results. Facial Plast Surg Clin North Am 2012;20(2):145–62.
9. Potter MJ, Harrison R, Ramsden A, et al. Facial acne and fine lines: transforming patient outcomes with plasma skin regeneration. Ann Plast Surg 2007;58(6):608–13.
10. Kono T, Groff WF, Sakurai H, et al. Treatment of traumatic scars using plasma skin regeneration (PSR) system. Lasers Surg Med 2009;41(2):128–30.
11. Theppornpitak N, Udompataikul M, Chalermchai T, et al. Nitrogen plasma skin regeneration for the treatment of mild-to-moderate periorbital wrinkles: a prospective, randomized, controlled evaluator-blinded trial. J Cosmet Dermatol 2019;18(1):163–8.
12. Fitzpatrik R, Bernstein E, Iyer S, et al. A histopathologic evaluation of the Plasma Skin Regeneration System (PSR) versus a standard carbon dioxide resurfacing laser in an animal model. Lasers Surg Med 2008;40(2):93–9.
13. Holcomb JD, Schucker A. Helium plasma skin regeneration–evaluation of skin tissue effects in a porcine model and comparison to nitrogen plasma skin regeneration. (Abstract presented at American Society for Laser Medicine and Surgery 2019 Annual Meeting, Denver, Colorado, USA). March 27–31, 2019.
14. Holcomb JD. Erbium:yttrium aluminum garnet laser skin resurfacing. In: Truswell WH, editor. Chapter 6 in lasers and light, peels and abrasions. New York: Thieme Medical Publishers; 2016.
15. Walia S, Alster TS. Famciclovir prophylaxis of herpes simplex virus reactivation after laser skin resurfacing. Dermatol Surg 1999;25(3):242–6.
16. Walia S, Alster TS. Cutaneous CO2 laser resurfacing infection rate with and without prophylactic antibiotics. Dermatol Surg 1999;25(11):857–61.
17. West TB, Alster TS. Effect of pretreatment on the incidence of hyperpigmentation following cutaneous CO2 laser resurfacing. Dermatol Surg 1999;25(1):15–7.
18. Widgerow AD, Fabi SG, Pasestine RF, et al. Extracellular matrix modulation: optimizing skin care and rejuvenation procedures. J Drugs Dermatol 2016;15(4 Suppl):s63–71.
19. Burkhardt BR, Maw R. Are more passes better? Safety versus efficacy with the pulsed CO2 laser. Plast Reconstr Surg 1997;100(8):1531–4.
20. Weinstein C, Pozner J, Scheflan M. Combined erbium:YAG laser resurfacing and face lifting. Plast Reconstr Surg 2001;107(2):586–92.

# Pulsed and Fractionated Techniques for Helium Plasma Energy Skin Resurfacing

Richard D. Gentile, MD, MBA[a,b,]*, J.D. McCoy, NMD[c]

## KEYWORDS

- Helium plasma energy skin resurfacing • Techniques • Pulsed • Fractioned
- Renuvion J-plasma laser skin rejuvenation

## KEY POINTS

- Energy-based skin rejuvenation has, like other forms of aesthetic treatments, the capability of achieving desirable end results.
- These end results must be balanced with the degree and duration of morbidity, which affect recovery from treatment.
- Renuvion skin resurfacing protocols include a free hand approach and we describe our preferred approach of pulsing and fractionating the helium plasma resurfacing energy.

## ENERGY-BASED SKIN REJUVENATION

Energy-based skin rejuvenation/resurfacing uses various forms of energy delivery to produce heat in the epidermis and dermis, in a controlled dose-dependent fashion. Heat produced from treatment can allow for precision tissue ablation or subablative changes with inflammatory remodeling of the reticular dermis, while limiting collateral thermal damage. The ideal outcome from energy delivery is a safe wound healing response with remodeling of tissue that improves a multitude of age-related changes: dyschromia, rhytides, elastosis/sagging, hydration, pore size, texture, and potentially volume loss. A new option for ablative skin rejuvenation Renuvion (Apyx Medical, Clearwater, Florida) was introduced in 2012. This device operates with a proprietary balance of helium plasma and radiofrequency (RF) and, unlike many skin rejuvenation devices that operate under pulsed duration exposures, the Renuvion can be used in continuous painting mode or intermittent pulsed technique mode. This article discusses a pulsed technique option for using Renuvion for ablative skin rejuvenation that the senior author (RDG) has developed and used since 2016 exclusively for his Renuvion skin rejuvenation patients. The options for fractionating the energy coming from this device also are reviewed in a technical description.

## METHODS OF ENERGY-BASED SKIN REJUVENATION

The market for nonsurgical, energy-based facial rejuvenation techniques has increased exponentially since lasers were first used for skin rejuvenation in 1983 and the concept of selective photothermolysis was presented.[1] Advances in this area have led to a wide range of devices that require the modern facial plastic surgeon to have a large repertoire of knowledge. Three broad categories of technology are leading non–energy-based rejuvenation technology: lasers, light therapy, and non–laser-based thermal tightening devices. Laser light therapy has continued to

facialplastic.theclinics.com

[a] Facial Plastic Surgery, Gentile Facial Plastic Surgery and Aesthetic Laser Center, 821 Kentwood Suite C, Youngstown, OH 44512, USA; [b] Facial Plastic Surgery, Cleveland Clinic Akron General Hospital, Akron, OH, USA; [c] Aesthetic Medicine, Contour Medical, 3345 S. Val Vista Drive, Suite 103, Gilbert, AZ 85297, USA
* Corresponding author. 821 Kentwood Suite C, Youngstown, OH 44512.
*E-mail address:* dr-gentile@msn.com

Facial Plast Surg Clin N Am 28 (2020) 75–85
https://doi.org/10.1016/j.fsc.2019.09.007
1064-7406/20/© 2019 Elsevier Inc. All rights reserved.

diversify with the use of ablative and nonablative resurfacing technologies, fractionated lasers, and their combined use. Broadband light (BBL) therapy has been developed for use in combination with other technologies or as a stand-alone technology. Finally, thermally based nonlaser skin-tightening devices, such as RF and intense focused ultrasonography, are evolving technologies that have changed rapidly over the past 5 years. Plasma technologies are new entries to the current assortment of devices and were introduced at the beginning of this millennium approximately 20 years ago. These devices use different media for plasma generation. including some using saline, but most plasma systems use noble gases for the purposes of ionization and plasma generation. Nitrogen plasma was introduced approximately 15 years ago[2,3] and Renuvion (helium/RF plasma) is the most recent plasma device introduced and was Food and Drug Administration approved in 2012.[4,5] Laser, light, RF, and plasma technologies represent an important advance in skin rejuvenation in the options for patients. Physical, technological, and clinical research currently is carried out in order to optimize energy device–skin interaction and energy device efficacy–safety profile. The different energy device sources are further summarized following the different spectral features of the laser sources used.[6]

UV laser and light sources have been used primarily for the treatment of inflammatory skin diseases and/or vitiligo as well as striae. The mechanism of action is immunomodulatory. The XeCl excimer laser emits at 308 nm, near the peak action spectrum for psoriasis. Other UV non-laser sources, like the 355nm, also have been used for vitiligo, hypopigmentation disorders, and various inflammatory diseases.

Violet intense pulsed light (IPL) spectra and low-power 410-nm light-emitting diode (LED) and fluorescent lamps both are used either alone or with aminolevulinic acid (ALA). Alone, the devices take advantage of endogenous porphyrins and kill *Propionibacterium acnes*. After application of ALA, this wavelength range is highly effective in creating singlet $O_2$ after absorption by *protoporphyrin IX*. Uses include treatment of actinic keratoses, actinic cheilitis, and basal cell carcinomas.

Near–infrared (IR)-A (595 nm, 755 nm, and 810 nm) wavelengths are used primarily to treat blood vessels and hyperpigmented lesions. They are positioned in the absorption spectrum for blood and melanin and penetrate deeply enough to treat vessels up to 2 mm. Newer lasers, such as the pulsed dye 595 nm, may be indicated for the treatment of port-wine stains and infantile hemangiomas. Quality (Q)-switched lasers in this spectrum may be useful to treat multicolored tattoos.

The 2 wavelengths, near–IR-B 940 nm and near–IR-B 1064 nm, have been used extensively for larger and deeper blood vessels on the legs and face. Because of the depth of penetration (on the order of millimeters), they are especially useful in coagulation of deeper blood vessels and selective follicle denaturation for safe and effective hair removal. Q-switched 1064-nm lasers are effective on dark ink tattoos.

Medium-IR lasers (1320–1540 nm) heat tissue water and shrink collagen and are widely used in cosmetology for antiaging purposes and treatment of striae and acne scarring (nonablative fractional procedures).

Far-IR systems are represented mainly by the $CO_2$ and Er:YAG lasers. Dermatologic applications are mainly surgical (warts and dermal nevi) and cosmetological, thanks to their precision in ablation. Fractional $CO_2$ lasers guarantee a precise epidermal and dermal heating that makes this device ideal for facial skin resurfacing (fine or moderate wrinkles, dyspigmentation, and acne scarring) on facial skin. Newer devices combine lasers with other energy sources, such as RF, in order to optimize antiaging dermatologic procedures.

Like any form of energy, RF devices, ablative RF or nonablative RF, have the capacity to produce heat—and although each brand-name application uses a slightly different technology, all work by resistive heating in the skin's deeper layers to induce new collagen and elastin production and encourage cell turnover, helping skin become firmer, thicker, and more youthful looking.

Sound is defined as mechanical energy that spreads through a medium in the form of waves. During ultrasound procedures, there typically is a gel that is placed on top of the skin that allows the sound waves to be sent through the gel to target different areas of the body. Ultrasound sends off sound waves that can cause vibrations. Depending on the frequency, these vibrations create heat within the body that can be tailored for different effects in the skin: the stimulation of collagen or the breakdown of adipose tissue.

In plasma devices, plasma skin regeneration technology uses energy delivered from plasma rather than light or RF only. Plasma typically is generated by an energy discharge, which can include RF, which causes ionization, excitation, or dissociation of gas or liquid molecules, leading to creation of various gaseous plasmas. The energy delivered produces a heating action that works at the skin's surface to remove old photo-damaged epidermal cells and below the skin surface or dermis to promote collagen growth.

## PRINCIPLES OF LASER AND ENERGY-BASED DEVICES FOR SKIN REJUVENATION

Laser is an acronym for light amplification by the stimulated emission of radiation. An understanding of the fundamental properties of laser light is essential to appreciate its clinical effects on the skin. First, laser light is monochromatic, meaning that the emitted light is composed of a single wavelength. Monochromatic light is determined by the medium of the laser system, through which the light passes. Second, laser light is coherent—traveling in phase spatially and temporally. Third, laser light is collimated—emitted in a parallel manner with minimal divergence. Laser light may be absorbed, reflected, transmitted, or scattered when applied to the skin. For a clinical effect to occur, light must be absorbed by tissue. Absorption of laser light is determined by chromophores—the target molecules found in the skin, which have specific wavelength absorption profiles. The 3 primary endogenous cutaneous chromophores are water, melanin, and hemoglobin, whereas tattoo ink represents an exogenous chromophore. On absorption of laser energy by the skin, photothermal, photochemical, or photomechanical effects may occur. The cutaneous depth of penetration of laser energy is dependent on absorption and scattering. In the epidermis, there is minimal light scattering, whereas in the dermis there is significant scatter due to the high concentration of collagen fibers. The amount of scattering of laser energy is inversely proportional to the wavelength of light. The depth of laser energy increases with wavelength until the midinfrared region of the electromagnetic spectrum, at which point dermal penetration becomes more superficial due to increased absorption within tissue water. The theory of selective photo thermolysis, proposed by Anderson and Parrish[1] in 1983, has been pivotal in the advancement of laser surgery. It explains the mechanism by which controlled destruction of a cutaneous target can be achieved without significant injury to surrounding tissue. Three principles are crucial to the process. First, an appropriate wavelength should be used that can be absorbed preferentially by the targeted tissue chromophore. Second, the pulse duration of the laser must be shorter than the chromophore's thermal relaxation time, which is the time required for the target to lose half of its peak temperature after irradiation. Third, the fluence (or energy) must be sufficient to achieve destruction of the target within the appropriate time interval. These factors guide the selection of lasers and IPL appropriate for a specific skin target or lesion. Lasers can be classified further by their mode of light emission. Continuous wave (CW) lasers produce a continuous beam of light with long exposure durations that can cause nonselective tissue damage. Quasi-CW mode produces interrupted emissions of constant laser energy by shuttering the CW beam into short intervals. Pulsed laser systems emit high-energy laser light in ultrashort pulse durations with relatively long interpulse time intervals. They can be long pulsed or very short pulsed, such as the Q-switched nanosecond and picosecond laser systems. IPL is a nonlaser filtered flash lamp device. Unlike lasers, IPL devices emit polychromatic, noncoherent, and noncollimated light (420–1400 nm) with varying pulse durations. The wider range of light can be absorbed by a variety of chromophores, making IPL less selective than lasers. As such, cutoff filters often are used to narrow the spectrum of emitted wavelengths and render the device more specific. Skin rejuvenation devices have been operated primarily in pulsed mode. The Renuvion device is one that can be operated in both continuous mode and pulsed mode. The origin of pulsing in skin rejuvenation was developed to be able to reach certain ablation thresholds for skin rejuvenation. Pulsed operation of lasers and energy devices refers to any device not classified as CW, so that the optical power appears in pulses of some duration at some repetition rate. This encompasses a wide range of technologies addressing several different motivations. Some lasers are pulsed simply because they cannot be run in continuous mode. In other cases, the application requires the production of pulses having as large an energy as possible. Because the pulse energy is equal to the average power divided by the repetition rate, this goal sometimes can be satisfied by lowering the rate of pulses so that more energy can be built up in between pulses. In laser ablation for example, a small volume of material at the surface of a work piece can be evaporated if it is heated in a very short time, whereas supplying the energy gradually would allow for the heat to be absorbed into the bulk of the piece, never attaining a sufficiently high temperature at a particular point. Other applications rely on the peak pulse power (rather than the energy in the pulse), especially to obtain nonlinear optical effects. For a given pulse energy, this requires creating pulses of the shortest possible duration using techniques, such as Q-switching. The optical bandwidth of a pulse cannot be narrower than the reciprocal of the pulse width. In cases of extremely short pulses, that implies lasing over a considerable bandwidth, contrary to the very narrow bandwidths typical of CW lasers. The lasing medium in some dye lasers and vibronic solid-state lasers produces optical gain over a wide bandwidth, making a laser possible, which can thus generate pulses of light as short as a few femtoseconds. In the Renuvion plasma device, very high energies and temperatures are generated by the helium ionization, and having adequate temperatures and energy for skin rejuvenation treatment is not a problem or a reason to suggest pulsing, but, to the contrary, pulsing is recommended to reduce excessive energy applied by the continuous-flow, freehand technique, which has been classically taught. A comparison of the reduced energies is discussed.

## HISTORY AND EVOLUTION OF PLASMA-BASED SKIN REJUVENATION

Plasma skin regeneration devices were introduced approximately 20 years ago and use a handpiece that has an ultra–high-frequency generator. The generator also can be in the electrosurgical unit (**Fig. 1** [Bovie Ultimate]). The generator energizes an inert gas (nitrogen for the original Portrait device or helium in the case of the Renuvion) so that its atoms and molecules separate (called ionization) into negatively charged electrons and positively charged ions. So, the inert gas becomes an activated ionized gas called plasma. Then millisecond pulses of plasma are sent to the skin via the handpiece. As the plasma hits the skin, there is an immediate energy transfer to the skin. The longer the pulse, the more energy delivered. Nitrogen plasma was the first gaseous plasma to be utilized for skin rejuvenation and or skin tightening and there are many publications on the safety and efficacy. When introduced, nitrogen plasma skin regeneration was a novel method of skin renewal that uses gaseous diatomic molecular nitrogen as an extracorporeal intermediary and energy reservoir to transduce RF energy in the device

handpiece just before delivery in alternate form (nitrogen plasma) to the skin's surface in a noncontact fashion. The nitrogen plasma energy is rapidly transferred to the skin's surface architecture, with gradient heating of deeper structures via thermal conduction. This creates a dual zone of injury with an outer (superficial) zone of irreversible thermal damage and an inner (deeper) zone of thermal modification.[2,3] Contrary to laser physics and the doctrine of selective photothermolysis, discussed previously,[1] nitrogen and helium plasma tissue interaction is non–chromophore dependent and is characterized by controlled predictable energy delivery to the skin's architecture, while at some settings and delivery methods avoiding certain phenomena (including excessive collateral thermal injury) often associated with ablative (chromophore dependent) laser tissue interaction. In further contrast to ablative lasers, the old skin architecture remains intact immediately after nitrogen plasma skin regeneration; there is no open wound. Neoepithelialization is rapid and generally complete within 5 days to 7 days after treatment. The old skin architecture serves as a protective biologic dressing and undergoes gradual desquamation as the neoepidermis appears.[2,3] As discussed previously, Renuvion or J-Plasma (Apyx Medical), for noncosmetic indications, uses helium gas, which is passed over the energized electrode; helium plasma is generated, which enables heat to be applied to tissue in 2 distinct modes. First, top-down non–chromophore-dependent thermal transfer occurs from the flowing hot helium gas occurs, with heat generated by the actual production of the plasma beam itself through the ionization and rapid neutralization of the helium atoms. The neutralization of the helium atoms gives rise to the characteristic violet optical emission (Lewis-Raleigh afterglow). Second, because plasmas are good electrical conductors, a portion of the RF energy used to energize the electrode and generate the plasma passes from the electrode to the tissue. An electrical displacement current is formed in the tissue

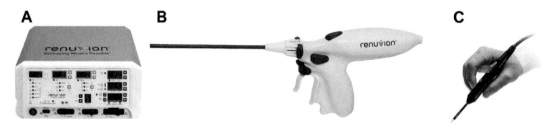

**A**        **B**                                          **C**

**Fig. 1.** (*A*) Renuvion generator cutting, coagulation, bipolar, and helium plasma. (*B*) Renuvion handpiece without generator. (*C*) J-Plasma handpiece with built-in generator. (*Courtesy of* Apyx Medical, Clearwater, FL; with permission.)

region immediately surrounding the helium plasma beam contact point both across the tissue surface and in depth. In 1 half-cycle, current flows into this region, accumulating charge that is withdrawn in the next half-cycle. The flow of current through the resistance of the tissue creates Joule (resistive) heating. So, the total energy applied by the RF component is added to the energy transfer noted by the ionization process and direct thermal transfer, a process known as instant tissue heating. The ionized or excited gaseous molecules, atoms, and even photons interact with the target tissue, which results in generation of surface-reactive species with biological potential, thermal heating, molecule scission, or even creation of secondary species/photons.[7,8] Consequently, these species or better said plasma-surface interactions cause damage at observed treated skin tissue. Damages caused are thermal injuries and UV radiation damages or result from the generation of reactive gaseous species, such as reactive oxygen species, reactive nitrogen species, or jointly named reactive oxygen and nitrogen species (RONS).[7,8] Furthermore, skin damage depends highly on different types of plasmas used and a variety of other parameters, such as a skin structure, the dosage of the plasma species, the exposure time to the treatment, and so forth. Hence, it also is essential to identify the boundaries of plasma toxicity to the skin after the treatment. With increasing flow rates, the temperature on treated skin rises and the gaseous RONS formation also increases as well as streamer formation. This results in direct skin damage and, unlike nitrogen plasma resurfacing, the helium plasma (Renuvion) usually does not have its thermal effects with an intact epidermis. These treatment effects more closely resemble a full-face ablative carbon dioxide laser treatment with eschar formation, which is wiped prior to subsequent treatment (**Fig. 2**).

## COMPARISON OF ENERGY LOAD: PULSED VERSUS CONTINUOUS HELIUM PLASMA SKIN REJUVENATION

The high-energy output of the Renuvion helium plasma device, which is due to instant tissue heating plus resistive heating of current formation, gives rise to the question of how much energy is needed to provide a superior clinical result versus what amount of energy does not result in additional clinical improvement but only additional morbidity. To understand the inherent energy load, the authors and associates have calculated the energy output and power output of various treatment options available with the Renuvion device. In these calculations, the amount of energy

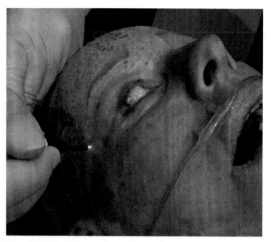

**Fig. 2.** Ablation eschar of epidermis with Renuvion pulsed helium plasma.

delivered to a fixed surface area of a 4-cm × 4-cm treated area is dependent on the treatment speed and the number of treatment lines needed to fully cover the area. The following calculations are an estimate and are based on assumptions on treatment technique. First is assuming a treatment speed of 1 cm/s when the treatment hand delivers the treatment.

- Based on a treatment speed of 1 cm/s, it takes 4 seconds to make 1 complete treatment line across the 4-cm × 4-cm square.
- Assume each treatment line is 3 mm or 0.3 cm wide.
- Based on a treatment line width of 0.3 cm, 13.33 complete treatment lines are needed to cover a 4-cm × 4-cm area—4 cm/0.3 cm per treatment line = 13.33 treatment lines.
- Multiply the number of treatment lines by the time it takes to make 1 treatment line to get the total activation time to cover a 4-cm × 4-cm area—4 seconds per treatment line × 13.33 treatment lines = 53.32 seconds of activation to cover a 4-cm × 4-cm square.
- Multiply the activation time of 53.32 seconds by the power output to get the Joules of energy delivered to a 4-cm × 4-cm section of tissue.
- The amount of energy delivered to a 4-cm × 4-cm treatment square for each setting scenario, described previously, is as follows:
  ○ 40%/4 L/min continuous—53.32 s × 6.575 J/s = 350.58 J
  ○ 40%/4 L/min 400 ms/200 ms pulsed – 53.32 s × 4.075 J/s = 217.28 J
  ○ 40%/4 L/min 200 ms/200 ms pulsed – 53.32 s × 3.225 J/s = 171.96 J

**Table 1**
**Comparison of energy load: pulsed versus continuous helium plasma skin rejuvenation**

| Generator Power Setting (%) | Helium Flow Rate (lpm) | Energy Mode | Pulsing Parameters | Energy Output (J) | Power Output (W or J/s) |
|---|---|---|---|---|---|
| 40 | 4 | Continuous | NA | 263 ± 13 | 6.575 |
| 40 | 4 | Pulsed | 400 ms on/200 ms off | 163 ± 13 | 4.075 |
| 40 | 4 | Pulsed | 200 ms on/200 ms off | 129 ± 7 | 3.225 |
| 40 | 4 | Pulsed | 100 ms on/200 ms off | 46 ± 7 | 1.15 |

     ○ 40%/4 L/min 100 ms/200 ms pulsed – 53.32 s × 1.15 J/s = 61.32 J (**Table 1**)

These calculations are completed in order to determine whether or not the pulsed technique delivers less energy than the continuous technique as a first step in answering, What is the best way to deliver the optimal dose of energy for optimal skin improvement without increasing morbidity by delivering more energy than necessary? The energy and power output of various modes of energy application are depicted in **Table 1**. The senior author (RDG) has always used a pulsed approach for Renuvion resurfacing in efforts to limit collateral tissue damage and prolonged recovery. The pulsed options may deliver shorter recoveries but an expedited recovery time would need to be determined by a randomized comparison of similar clinical conditions treated by each of the study parameters. Some clinical anecdotal observations also may be noted as well as the prevalence or absence of complications regarding each treatment paradigm. The pulsed technique used by the author usually is preceded by a single ablation pass, of 100-um passes of Renuvion Er:YAG. One pass or 2 passes of Renuvion, at 40% 4 L/min and 400 ms/200 ms, are completed. Second passes are done only on the most severely sun-damaged and wrinkled skin.

## FRACTIONATING RENUVION HELIUM PLASMA ENERGIES

In a further effort to reduce the significant energies delivered by both the continuous and pulsed ablation modes, the author sought to develop a fractionating option. Although different approaches are in consideration for fractionating helium plasma energy, the author selected a heat-resistant grid (**Fig. 3**) to use in order to block out much of the energy seen by delivering a continuous or pulsed mode treatment. The grid utilized is a high heat–resistant silicone grid and, when used in conjunction with the flame of the plasma plume, the result is a clearly fractionated ablation zone (**Fig. 4**) The

fractionating of the helium plasma is done in more heat-sensitive areas, such as the periorbital region, and is used a partial treatment pass if 1 pass has already been given. Like pulsing, the fractionating of the plasma plume can serve to limit the excess energy that can be possible with continuous or high-density pulsed exposures. An estimate of the reduction in energy seen in fractionated patients seems to be from 20% to 40% of what is seen in the continuous and pulsed modes. More studies on the energy output of different treatment protocols will be helpful in determining the precise degree of energy reduction for this new technology. On the fractionated grid, the continuous mode is used at 40% power and 4 L/min.

## HELIUM PLASMA (RENUVION) SKIN REJUVENATION, CONTINUOUS METHOD

All continuous mode cases were done exclusively using an ionized helium gas plasma device (Renuvion/J-plasma) using continuous flow of helium gas, at 4-L flow, and various power settings, ranging from 10% to 40% power. Even in continuous flow (ie, nonpulsed), the ionization of helium

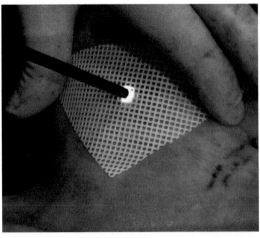

**Fig. 3.** Silicone fractionating grid used with Renuvion skin rejuvenation, continuous mode, 40% and 4 L.

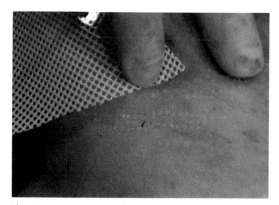

**Fig. 4.** Appearance of fractional plasma ablation zones obtained with fractionating grid.

from the RF generator is biphasic, so it is technically not 100% continuous. Pretreatment, 3-dimensional photos of patients are taken (Vectra H1 [Canfield Scientific, Parsippany, NJ, USA]), with an hour consult to review day of treatment, medication history, prescriptions (antiviral, steroidal, and antibiotic), and post-treatment protocols. Immediately before treatment, patients are prepped with topical anesthetic (lidocaine, prilocaine, and phenylephrine, 10% / 10% / 1%, apply to lidocaine, prilocaine, and phenylephrine [combination]) for 30 minutes and for oral anxiolysis with 0.25-mg to 0.5-mg triazolam, cleansed, and degreased, and grounding pad is applied. Supraorbital, supratrochlear, infraorbital, zygomatic, and mental blocks are performed (lidocaine 1% with epinephrine and bicarbonate buffer). Low-

volume Klein solution (lidocaine 0.2% with epinephrine and bicarbonate buffer; total 500 mL prepped) is used to tumesce the full face from the hairline to 1 thumb breadth below the mandible, using 22-gauge, 70 mm blunt-tipped cannula (Steriglide [TSK, Japan]).

Case 1 was a 63-year old man with pervasive acne scarring. First-pass settings, of 4-L helium flow and 40% power, were to the full face, with only a single pass periorbitally, at 4-L flow and 20% power. Second pass, performed after gentle débridement of eschar from the full face (periorbital eschar was left intact), was at 4-L flow and 40% power. A third pass with minimal dwell was performed only over each deep scar, at 4-L flow and 20% power. Low-level LED (Celluma PRO, BioPhotas, Anaheim, California) was performed daily, starting 48 hours post-resurfacing for 10 days, and 1 BBL photofacial was performed with 560-nm filter 6 weeks post-resurfacing. No additional treatment was used in this case. Post-treatment photo is 8 months after resurfacing (**Fig. 5**).

Case 2 was a 61-year old woman with pervasive full-facial rhytides. First-pass settings, of 4-L helium flow and 40% power, were to the full face, with only a single pass periorbitally, at 4-L flow and 30% power. Second pass, after gentle débridement of eschar from the full face (periorbital eschar was left intact), was at 4-L flow and 40% power. Low-level LED (Celluma) was performed daily starting 48 hours post-resurfacing for 10 days, and 3 BBL photofacials were performed with a 560-nm filter at 6 weeks, 10 weeks, and

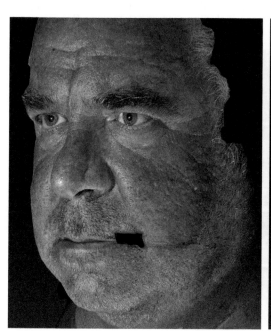
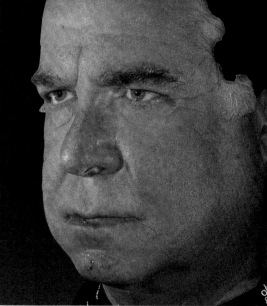

**Fig. 5.** Case study 1. (*Left*) Before Renuvion pulsed treatment. (*Right*) After Renuvion pulsed treatment.

20 weeks post-resurfacing. No additional treatment was used in this case. Post-treatment photo is 6 months after resurfacing (**Fig. 6**).

Case 3 was a 59-year old woman with deep perioral rhytides. First-pass settings, of 4-L flow and 35% power, were full face, with only a single pass periorbitally, at 4-L flow and 20% power. Second pass, after gentle débridement of eschar from full face (periorbital eschar was left intact), were at 4-L flow and 30% power. A third pass periorally, at 4-L flow and 20% power, produced full visual elimination of rhytides. Low-level LED (Celluma) was performed daily starting 48 hours post-resurfacing for 10 days, and 3 BBL photofacials were performed with 515 nm and 560 nm filters at 6 weeks, 11 weeks, and 15 weeks post-resurfacing. Post-treatment photo is 8 months after resurfacing.

In all cases, serially reduced power (40%, 30%, 20%, and 10%) from the second-pass power setting was used to blend to approximately 2 thumb breadths below the mandible. Post-treatment home care for all cases included multiple daily showers, use of Vaniply ointment (Pharmaceutical Specialties Inc., Rochester, MN), ASAP 20-ppm silver gel (20 ppm) (American Biotech Labs, American Fork, Utah), and Lasercyn hypochlorite spray, as needed. All cases were re-epithelialized within 10 days to 14 days, with varying erythema that persisted for 2 months to 4 months (**Fig. 7**).

## HELIUM PLASMA (RENUVION) SKIN REJUVENATION PULSED TECHNIQUE

In case studies, pulsed cases were performed using a combination of 2940-nm Er:Yag laser (Contour TRL [Sciton, Palo Alto, CA]) for initial pass and ionized helium gas plasma (Renuvion/J-Plasma) for all additional passes, in pulsed mode. With this technique, the erbium is used to precisely ablate 90 μm to 100 μm, without the necessity to débride the eschar before additional passes. After the first pass with erbium, ionized helium plasma can be delivered in a pulsed form, where the user dictates on/off time (eg, 200 ms on and 200 ms off). Depending on preferred technique, which includes a static point-to-point delivery or flowing brushstroke movement, users can dictate longer or shorter on times. Patient pretreatment consultation and treatment preparation are identical to continuous mode cases, discussed previously.

Case 4 was a 67-year old woman with dyschromia and fine rhytides. First-pass settings, of 100-μm ablation with 50% overlap Er:Yag, to the full face, excluding periorbital region. Second pass delivered ionized helium gas, in pulsed mode (400 ms on and 200 ms off), at 4-L flow and 30% power, to the full face, with only 1 pass periorbitally at the same pulsed setting. No eschar was removed periorbitally. Pulsed energy was delivered in motion. Low-level LED (Celluma) was performed daily starting 48 hours post-resurfacing for 10 days, and 3 BBL photofacials were performed with a 560-nm filter at 4 weeks, 8 weeks, and 12 weeks. Post-treatment photo is 6 months after resurfacing (**Fig. 8**).

Case 5 was a 59-year old woman with pervasive rhytides and laxity. First-pass settings, of 100-μm ablation with 50% overlap Er:Yag, to the full face, including periorbital region. Second pass

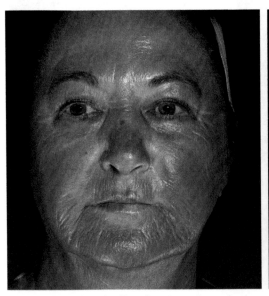
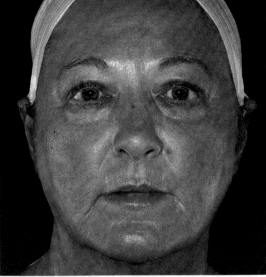

**Fig. 6.** Case study 2. (*Left*) Before Renuvion pulsed treatment. (*Right*) After Renuvion pulsed treatment.

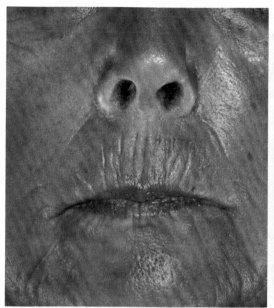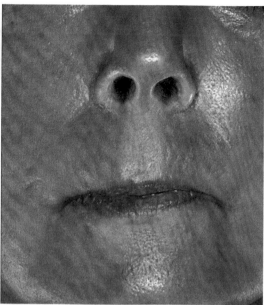

**Fig. 7.** Case study 3. (*Left*) Before Renuvion pulsed treatment. (*Right*) After Renuvion pulsed treatment.

delivered ionized helium gas, in pulsed mode (400 ms on and 200 ms off), at 4-L flow and 40% power, to the full face, with only 1 pass periorbitally at the same pulsed setting. No eschar was removed periorbitally. A third pass of ionized helium gas, in pulsed mode (400 ms on and 200 ms off), at 4-L flow and 40% power, was performed periorally and throughout the midface in the region of the most significant rhytides (**Fig. 9**).

Case 6 was a 63-year old woman with pervasive rhytides and laxity. First-pass settings, of 100-μm ablation with 50% overlap Er:Yag, to the full face, including periorbital region. Second pass delivered ionized helium gas, in pulsed mode (400 ms on, 200 ms off), at 4-L flow and 40% power, to the full face, with only 1 pass periorbitally at the same pulsed setting. No eschar was removed periorbitally. A third pass of ionized

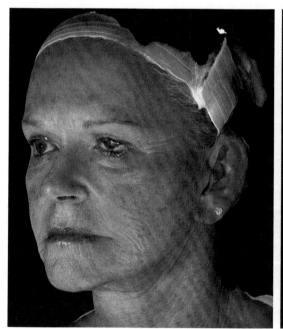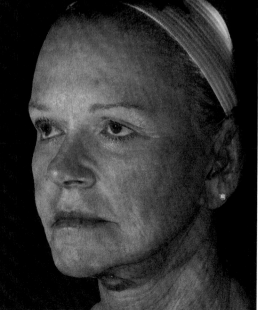

**Fig. 8.** Case study 4. (*Left*) Before Renuvion pulsed treatment. (*Right*) After Renuvion pulsed treatment.

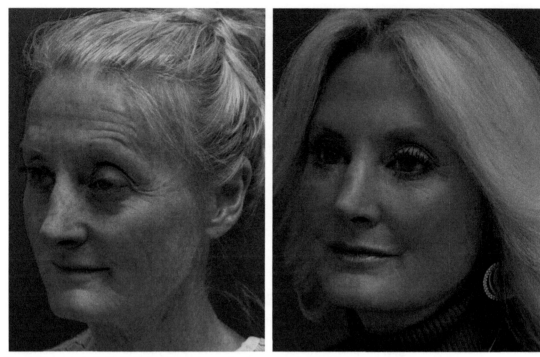

**Fig. 9.** Case study 5. (*Left*) Before Renuvion pulsed treatment. (*Right*) After Renuvion pulsed treatment.

helium gas, in pulsed mode (400 ms on and 200 ms off), at 4-L flow and 40% power, was performed periorally and throughout the midface in the region of the most significant rhytides (**Fig. 10**).

## HELIUM PLASMA (RENUVION) SKIN REJUVENATION: FRACTIONATED TECHNIQUE

Case 7 was a 67-year old woman with pervasive rhytides and laxity. First-pass settings, of 100-μm

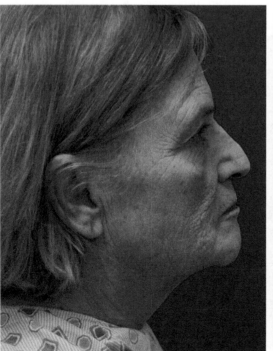
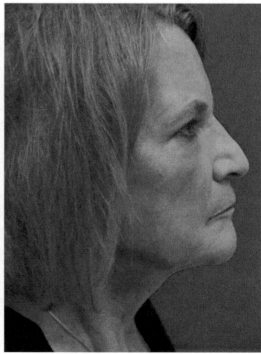

**Fig. 10.** Case study 6. (*Left*) Before Renuvion pulsed treatment. (*Right*) After Renuvion pulsed treatment.

A                              B

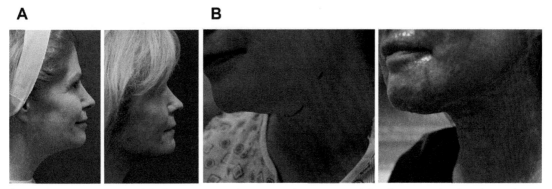

**Fig. 11.** Case study 7. (*A*) Left before Renuvion fractionated treatment. Right after Renuvion fractionated treatment. (*B*) Left and right before and after Renuvion fractionated treatment.

ablation with 50% overlap Er:Yag, to the full face, including periorbital region. Second pass delivered ionized helium gas, in continuous mode, over fractionating silicone grid, at 4-L flow and 40% power, to the full face, with only 1 pass periorbitally at the same pulsed setting. No eschar was removed periorbitally. A third pass of ionized helium gas, in pulsed mode (400 ms on and 200 ms off), at 4-L flow and 40% power, was performed periorally and throughout the midface (**Fig. 11**).

## SUMMARY

Energy-based skin rejuvenation has, like other forms of aesthetic treatments, the capability of achieving desirable end results. These end results must be balanced with degree and duration of morbidity, which affect recovery from treatment. After the Food and Drug Administration approval process, the settings and protocols for newly released devices are not always at the optimal settings due to lack of clinical experience with a new device. In some new technology introductions, the settings may be lower than what are eventually determined to be more optimal. In some new devices, the setting may involve more energy transfer than is necessary for satisfactory treatment. In efforts to achieve a satisfactory balance of energy applied, clinical results, and post-treatment morbidity and recovery, a protocol for reducing energy output by pulsing the plasma device rather than operating in continuous mode is presented. In addition, the authors have been pleased with using fractionating grids of thermal-resistant silicone to further reduce the excess energies associated with full-face plasma resurfacing with Renuvion in continuous mode. In balancing therapeutic results with the post-treatment recovery, the authors notice a reduction in recovery times for pulsed and fractionated

techniques, although the improvements in these parameters need to be subject to additional studies.

## DISCLOSURE

None.

## REFERENCES

1. Anderson RR, Parrish JA. Selective photothermolysis: precise microsurgery by selective absorption of pulsed radiation. Science 1983;220(4596):524–7.
2. Holcomb JD, Kent K, Rousso D. Nitrogen plasma skin regeneration and aesthetic facial surgery. multicenter evaluation of concurrent treatment. Arch Facial Plast Surg 2009;11(3):184–93.
3. Kilmer S, Semchyshyn N, Shah G, et al. A pilot study on the use of a plasma skin regeneration device (Portrait®PSR3) in full facial rejuvenation procedures. Lasers Med Sci 2007;22(2):101–9.
4. Gentile RD. Cool atmospheric plasma (J-Plasma) and new options for facial contouring and skin rejuvenation of the heavy face and neck. Facial Plast Surg 2018;34(1):66–74.
5. Gentile RD. Renuvion/J-plasma for subdermal skin tightening facial contouring and skin rejuvenation of the face and neck. Facial Plast Surg Clin North Am 2019;27(3):273–90.
6. Nistico SP, Chiricozzi A, Tamburi F, et al. Lasers and energy devices for the skin: conventional and unconventional use. Biomed Res Int 2016;2016: 9031091. Available at: https://www.hindawi.com/journals/bmri/2016/9031091/. Accessed June 1, 2019.
7. von Woedtke T, Metelmann HR, Weltmann KD. Clinical plasma medicine: state and perspectives of in vivo application of cold atmospheric plasma. J Wound Care 2018;27(Suppl 9):S4–10.
8. Kalghatgi S, Kelly CM, Cerchar E, et al. Effects of nonthermal plasma on mammalian cells. PLoS One 2011; 6(1):e16270.

# Picosecond Laser
## Tattoos and Skin Rejuvenation

Raminder Saluja, MD[a], Richard D. Gentile, MD, MBA[b,c],*

## KEYWORDS

- Picosecond • LIOB • Photomechanical effect • FOCUS lens • Skin revitalization • Picotoning

## KEY POINTS

- Picosecond laser technology uses ultra-short pulses in the trillionths of a second (10–12) creating photomechanical and photoacoustic effects on the skin.
- FOCUS lens is a diffractive lens array that creates high-powered microbeams per pulse and leads to the creation of light-induced optical breakdown (LIOB).
- The resultant skin effects from the creation of the LIOB are minimization of pigmentation and improvement of elastin and collagen.

## INTRODUCTION

Laser science is one of the most innovative fields in modern medicine. Discernible progression has occurred from early theoretic work by Townes in 1953 to present day laser science.[1,2] The application of laser science in the medical arena has expanded into a multitude of specialties including dermatology, plastic surgery, ophthalmology, urology, cardiology, orthopedics, etc.

The cornerstone of laser science begins with selective photothermolysis, described by Anderson and Parish.[3] When the targeted chromophore is irradiated by a preferentially absorbed wavelength at an energy setting capable of target destruction, delivered at pulse durations less then thermal relaxation times of the target, then the adjacent tissue is spared thus confining destruction to the target alone.[3] Application of this principle greatly minimizes nonselective thermal damage and enhances the precision of laser irradiation in achieving intended outcomes.

## PICOSECOND PULSE

A picosecond is defined as a pulse in the trillionths of a second ($10^{-12}$), whereas nanoseconds are pulsed in the billionths of a second ($10^{-9}$). Although both nanosecond and picosecond pulses can generate high target temperatures above steam formation, picosecond lasers have a faster rate of power delivery generating higher target pressure in the irradiated tissue with less thermal diffusion.

The initial cutaneous study evaluating the hypothesis that picosecond lasers were more effective than nanosecond pulses in clearing tattoos was conducted on 16 patients by Ross and colleagues[4] in 1998. Each tattoo was divided into 3 sections treated with an Nd:YAG picopulsed laser, nanosecond domain laser, or a control. All sections were evaluated with electron microscopy and assessed by blinded investigators. Most of the sections treated with the picopulsed laser (12/16 patients) displayed greater clearance of ink at lower energies and a greater depth of penetration when parameters were held constant.

In 1999 Herd[5] performed a comparative split study with a picopulsed laser and nanosecond laser on 6 albino guinea pigs and concluded that the picosecond laser was more effective than nanosecond laser in clearing tattoo pigment. Computer simulations have confirmed that high target

[a] Saluja Cosmetic and Laser Center, Private Practice, 9615 Northcross Center Court, Suite B, Huntersville, NC 28078, USA; [b] Facial Plastic Surgery, Gentile Facial Plastic Surgery and Aesthetic Laser Center, 821 Kentwood Suite C, Youngstown, OH 44512, USA; [c] Cleveland Clinic Akron General Hospital, Akron, OH, USA
* Corresponding author. Facial Plastic Surgery, Gentile Facial Plastic Surgery and Aesthetic Laser Center, 821 Kentwood Suite C, Youngstown, OH 44512.
*E-mail address:* dr-gentile@msn.com

Facial Plast Surg Clin N Am 28 (2020) 87–100
https://doi.org/10.1016/j.fsc.2019.09.008
1064-7406/20/© 2019 Elsevier Inc. All rights reserved.

pressures generated with picosecond pulses lead to high peak tensile stress that fragment ink particles via a photomechanical impact, not previously seen with nanosecond pulses.[6] Particle fragmentation created by picosecond pulses was described at ASLMS 2013[7] as linearly dependent on laser fluence and quadratically dependent on pulse duration. With a short pulse duration, a higher photomechanical impact is imparted on ink particles, exceeding the tissue's threshold, leading to greater efficacy in particle fragmentation.[8]

## PicoSure

In 2012, PicoSure brand laser system (Hologic-Cynosure, Westford, MA, USA) emerged as the first commercially available picosecond laser receiving Food and Drug Administration (FDA) clearance for cutaneous use (**Fig. 1**). The solid state, alexandrite laser, is equipped with a zoom optic allowing for titratable changes in spot size and fluence through a rotational movement on the handpiece and can deliver up to 200mj/pulse. In addition, there are 3 separate handpieces (6 mm, 8 mm, and 10 mm), equipped with either a flat or a diffractive lens array for the treatment of benign pigmentation, acne scarring, striae, and rhytides. Additional wavelengths (532 nm, 1064 nm) have been added to the PicoSure workstation to further expand capabilities in treating red, yellow, and orange ink.

## TATTOO

Tattooing has been performed since prehistoric times and the word "tattoo" is derived from the Polynesian word "tatau" brought to Europe by Captain Cook after visiting Tahiti.[9] Tattoos are categorized as cosmetic, traumatic, decorative, or medical and involve the application of ink percutaneously placed into the papillary dermis. A portion of the ink may descend into the reticular dermis and blur the tattoo or may partially fragment via the immune system and clear intrinsically. In the past, a multitude of destructive techniques were used for tattoo removal, including mechanical abrasive techniques, surgical excision, and ablative techniques, each creating its own subset of adverse events.

Nanosecond laser technology, using principles of selective photothermolysis[3] heralded a new era of targeting and removing ink; however, multiple treatments were needed and dyspigmentation, textural irregularity, and stagnant, residual ink known as a "recalcitrant tattoo" would still occur. As ink particle size diminishes, a higher impact is needed for additional fragmentation. To achieve

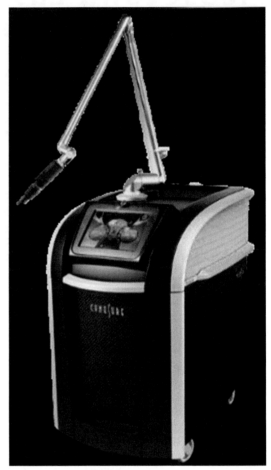

**Fig. 1.** PicoSure laser with zoom optic. (*Courtesy of Cynosure, Westford, MA; with permission.*)

this, higher fluence parameters were selected to create additional fragmentation while often times crossing the threshold of cutaneous safety.

Sub-nanosecond pulses deliver both photothermal and photomechanical stress to shatter the target before any substantial thermal dispersion can occur to the tissue, thus aiding the safety profile while improving efficacy. An initial study done by Brauer and colleagues[10] evaluated blue and green tattoos, traditionally difficult colors to clear, with a 750 to 900 picosecond laser prototype and found 75% clearance in 11/12 tattoos with 1 to 2 treatments. A second study performed by Saedi and colleagues[11] confirmed the efficiency of the laser with 75% reduction of ink in 2 to 4 treatments. In the clinic, the authors have seen reduction of green ink even with minimal treatments (**Fig. 2**).

The addition of the frequency-doubled Nd:YAG of 532 nm wavelength, which received FDA clearance in 2015, increased capabilities to treat red, orange, and yellow dye. In vitro studies have

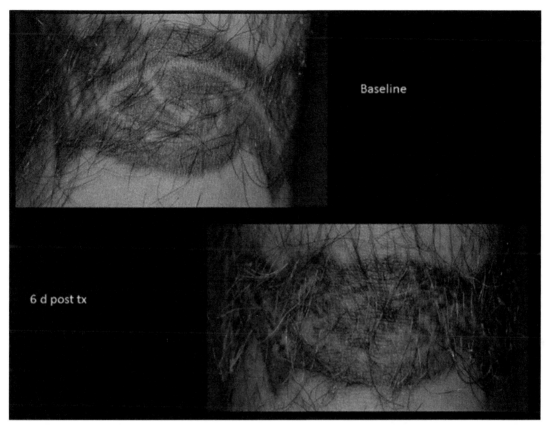

**Fig. 2.** Six days after 1 treatment with PicoSure. (*Courtesy of* Cynosure, Westford, MA.)

demonstrated the peak absorption wavelengths of yellow tattoo ink measures at 440 nm and 470 to 485 nm, which are nonexistent with our current lasers.[12,13] Favorable outcomes with PicoSure 532 nm on yellow ink were published, and the investigators concluded that yellow dye may be more susceptible to the photomechanical impact imparted on the ink.[14] In 2016, the 1064 nm wavelength was added to the platform.

Sub-nanosecond pulses exert a combination of effects starting with photothermal expansion that creates high tensile stress on the target. This subsequently causes photomechanical fragmentation leading to a photoacoustic "pop" that reverberates in the tissue as a shock wave.[15] With respect to ultra-short pulses, the peak tensile strength or the ability to disrupt the target is achieved with much lower fluences than comparative nanosecond technology.

Tattoo pigments have particle sizes ranging from 40 to 300 nm, which correspond to thermal relaxation times in the picosecond range (estimated 12–1060 picoseconds).[16]

**Fig. 3** shows a distal appendage tattoo (finger) that was previously treated with nanosecond lasers until clearance plateau. The tattoo was then treated with PicoSure and the residual ink cleared.

## LASER TATTOO CONSULT

During consultation, the authors follow the Kirby Desai[17] checklist. They begin by documenting the Fitzpatrick skin type of the patient. Although practitioners have treated darker Fitzpatrick skin types, the authors recommend test spotting Fitz IV and higher if using 755 nm and typically revert to 1064 nm for patients with Fitz V and VI skin type.

The authors indicate if the tattoo is professionally placed or is an amateur tattoo, as the latter typically has less ink density and ink placement may be more superficial, lending itself to quicker clearance.

The age of the tattoo is documented, as fading can intrinsically occur over time. The authors evaluate for scarring in the area, as this may lead to laser light scatter and an immune blockade that may minimize clearance, although they have noted clearance of tattoo ink and even improvement of baseline scarring when treated with PicoSure

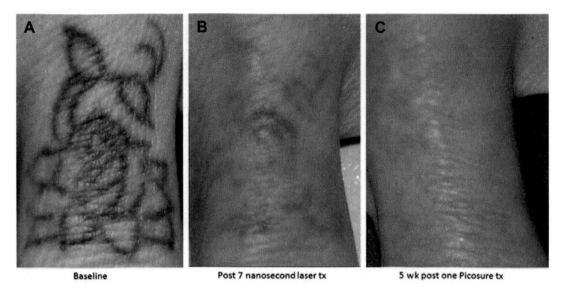

| Baseline | Post 7 nanosecond laser tx | 5 wk post one Picosure tx |

**Fig. 3.** Recalcitrant finger tattoo. After 1 PicoSure treatment. (*A*) Baseline. (*B*) After 7 nanosecond lasers. (*C*) Five weeks after 1 PicoSure laser. (*Courtesy of* Cynosure, Westford, MA.)

(**Fig. 4**). They also document if the patient is a smoker, or has poor health, which may slow clearance.

It is important to indicate if the tattoo is covering another smaller tattoo, and if so, document the colors of the hidden tattoo.

The location of the tattoo is important, as head and neck locations have an abundance of regional lymph nodes and vascular supply facilitating clearance while areas such as the distal appendages pose the greatest challenge for clearance.

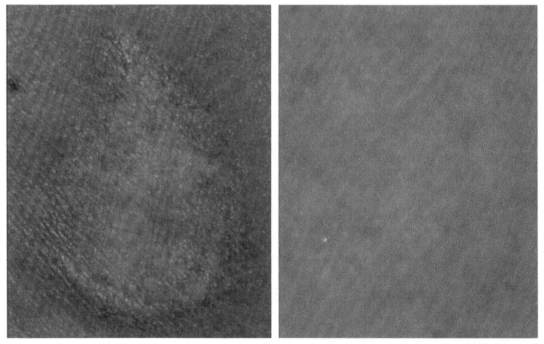

**Fig. 4.** (*Left*) Iridescent blue tattoo on neck with baseline fibrotic ridge of scarring inferiorly. (*Right*) After 9 PicoSure laser Tx with clearance of ink and improvement of baseline scarring. (*Courtesy of* Cynosure, Westford, MA.)

The process can be painful. Topical numbing can be used for smaller tattoos as the risk of lidocaine toxicity should be respected. Subcutaneous lidocaine injection is not recommended secondary to increased risk of scarring and laser light scatter. Cold air or ice may also minimize discomfort.

Immediately after treatment a low-powered, low pulse duration fractional $CO_2$ laser may be used to create fractional zones, as an egress pathway for fluid helps hasten healing.

Ointment-based emollients are recommended for 4 days posttreatment, and patients are recommended to keep the area out of stagnant water (hot tubs, pools, soaking in bath tub). The treatments are separated by 10 to 12 weeks. Strict sun protection is followed pre- and posttreatment to avoid pigmentary issues.

## FOCUS LENS ARRAY

The FOCUS lens is a hexagonal lens array etched with a diffractive grating on the refracting surface (**Fig. 5**). This specially designed lens minimizes aberrations to improve the optical performance. The lens is equipped with a 25 mm spacer and delivers 70% of the total emitted energy to the underlying skin through high-intensity microbeams.[18] The remaining 30% of energy is emitted at the lower fluence associated with each of the tips (6 mm = 0.71 j/cm$^2$, 8 mm = 0.4 j/cm$^2$, and 10 mm = 0.25 J/cm$^2$). As the spot size increases, the number of microbeams increase, which minimizes the energy output per microbeam.

The pitch between the centers of each microbeam is 500 microns. Per pulse, up to 10% of the underlying tissue is exposed to the higher-energy microbeams allowing multiple passes to be delivered while protecting the skin from a full-field, higher fluence setting. Although the 6 mm FOCUS lens is used routinely in Fitzpatrick skin types I to III, a larger spot size of 8 mm or 10 mm, with associated lower fluences, may be used for Fitz IV and V.

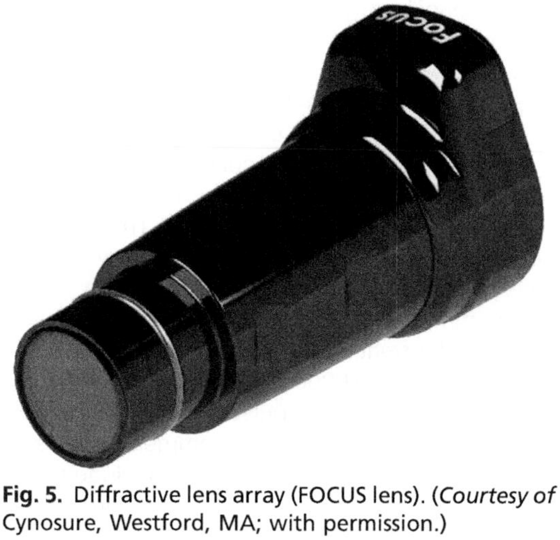

## LIGHT-INDUCED OPTICAL BREAKDOWN

A light-induced optical breakdown (LIOB) is the unique histologic finding that occurs with the diffractive lens array in the epithelial layer. Photo-thermo-mechanical disruption is the initiator of the LIOB.[19] Melanosomes and melanin granules absorb the picosecond photons, which are pulsed in shorter durations, then the thermal relaxation time of the granules. Melanin granules become "superheated" and behave as a nucleation site for microbubble formation. These spatially separated microbubbles coalesce, increase in size, and finally collapse, dissipating their energy through shock wave emission.[20]

Tanghetti describes this phenomenon histologically as an intraepidermal injury surrounded by unaltered appearing cells with an intact overlying stratum corneum. The high-energy microbeams are readily absorbed by melanin leading to ionization (ejection of a free electron). The free electrons continue to increase in an avalanche style process, blocking the microbeam from propagating any further than the epithelial melanin. The laser beam terminates and creates an intraepidermal, spherical vacuole or LIOB at the termination location (**Fig. 6**), visualized within minutes of laser irradiation.[18,20] At 24 hours, the vacuole is filled with rehydrated cellular debris staining positively for melanin (**Fig. 7**). The vacuole contracts over the next days to weeks. Microscopic epidermal necrotic debris (MENDS) can also be visualized,

**Fig. 5.** Diffractive lens array (FOCUS lens). (*Courtesy of* Cynosure, Westford, MA; with permission.)

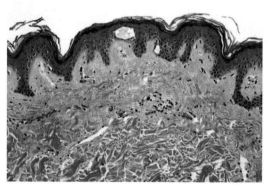

**Fig. 6.** Ten minutes posttreatment showing focal injuries in epidermis (LIOB). (*Courtesy of* E. Tanghetti, MD; with permission.)

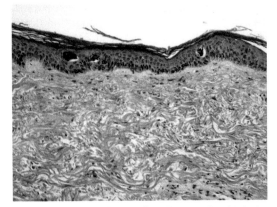

**Fig. 7.** Twenty-four hours after showing focal injuries with vacuole filled with cellular debris. (*Courtesy of* E. Tanghetti, MD; with permission.)

which exfoliates between 3 and 5 weeks posttreatment. The combination of debris-filled vacuoles and MENDS help to shunt and clear unwanted pigmentation.

Dermal inflammation is visualized after 24 hours (**Fig. 8**) and is thought to be caused by microbubble formation and photoacoustic interactions sending pressure waves into the dermis. McDaniel has shown how direct exposure to fibroblasts with an alexandrite wavelength causes changes in cell signaling and cytokine release from alterations in cellular membranes. Upregulation of heat shock proteins was noted leading to increased collagen and elastin with downregulation of elastinase.[21] McDaniel continued exploring his hypothesis by showing histologic evidence of new collagen and elastin in the dermis 3 and 6 months after FOCUS lens treatment.

Dermal remodeling via FOCUS lens represents a new method in rebuilding dermal architecture not

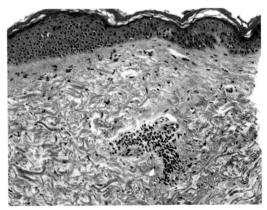

**Fig. 8.** Healing response in dermis, after 24 hours leading to new collagen and elastin. (*Courtesy of* E. Tanghetti, MD; with permission.)

solely reliant on thermal mechanisms. Although thermal methods are involved, they are occurring more at the granular level of the chromophore (melanin), which initiates the subsequent photomechanical and photoacoustic processes. The melanin index of the skin should be taken into consideration when selecting laser parameters.

## ACNE SCARRING—FDA CLEARED JULY 2014

Brauer and colleagues[22] did a study evaluating the FOCUS lens in 20 acne scarred patients with Fitzpatrick skin types II to V. Six treatments were performed every 4 to 8 weeks. A 3-dimensional scar analysis revealed a mean 24.3% improvement, maintained at 1 (24.0%) and 3 (27.2%) months after treatment. Histologic analysis revealed elongation and increased density of elastic fibers, with an increase in dermal collagen and mucin. In addition, reduction in residual postinflammatory hyperpigmentation was visualized. This remains the treatment of choice when treating acne scarring in adolescent patients with associated PIH (**Fig. 9**).

## PROCEDURE FOR ACNE SCARRING

After the face is thoroughly cleansed, topical numbing can be applied (optional). Treatment begins with one quadrant at a time and multiple passes are placed until confluent erythema is achieved. Posttreatment patients will feel heat effects for 1 to 3 hours. Higher melanin index patients will experience erythema quicker with lower total pulses. Lower fluences are used with Fitzpatrick skin types IV through VI. Perioral edema will be noted for 1 to 4 hours posttreatment, and some patients may experience a papillary type of response that may be secondary to a histamine release or vascular interaction in lower melanin index patients. The LIOB created in patients with melanin index of 12 or lower may contain a combination of melanin and red blood cells.[23] If this occurs, antihistamine taken 1 hour before subsequent treatments may help. Three to six treatments are recommended every 4 to 6 weeks.

Recommended pulse counts with the diffractive lens array for treating acne scarring, full-face acne is between 3000 to 6000 pulses. A small pilot study evaluated standard pulse recommendation compared with higher than recommended pulses in a split face design. The study concluded that additional pulses greater than the standard protocol did not yield statistically significant

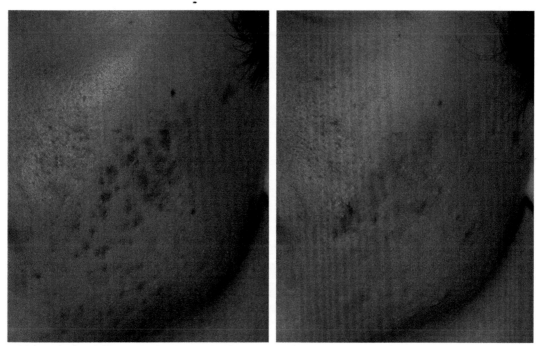

**Fig. 9.** After 2 PicoSure 6 mm FOCUS lens with improvement in PIH and texture. PIH, postinflammatory hyperpigmentation. (*Courtesy of* Cynosure, Westford, MA.)

improvement but also did not cause an increase in side effects other than transient increases in erythema and mild edema.[24]

## SKIN REVITALIZATION—FDA CLEARED SEPTEMBER 2014

Because of the increased luminosity associated with the reduction of fine lines and wrinkles, the term "skin revitalization" was coined for this treatment. Weiss and colleagues completed a prospective, blinded study evaluating the efficacy and safety of the treatment of perioral and ocular wrinkles using the 6-mm diffractive lens with the 755 nm wavelength on 40 subjects with Fitzpatrick skin types I to IV. Subjects received 4 treatments monthly with an average of 5000 pulses delivered over 4 passes to the treatment site. In addition, 6 patients had biopsies performed at the treatment site for histologic evaluation.

A statistically significant reduction of rhytids was observed and histologic analysis confirmed an increased density and depth to the new dermal architecture visualized at 6 months. Most of the patients had edema and erythema resolving within hours. The reduction in benign pigmentation, added to the textural improvement constituted the "revitalization" properties seen in the skin posttreatment.[25]

## PICOTONING

Laser toning had traditionally been performed with a Q-switched neodymium-doped yttrium aluminum garnet laser and had gained popularity for facial rejuvenation in the Asian population.[26,27] Multiple treatments were required for visual results. Even at subselective photothermolytic settings, issues such as leucoderma, postinflammatory hyperpigmentation, and generalized rebound pigmentation could occur.

Conceptually, using a picosecond laser, with less thermal effects, could provide an alternative to higher Fitzpatrick skin patients with benign pigmentation, by targeting melanin at lower fluences, thereby minimizing secondary pigmentary alterations. Picotoning summarizes the cutaneous changes induced by FOCUS lens by targeting unwanted pigmentation while improving the texture and tone to the skin through new collagen and elastin production.

The clinical results of the FOCUS lens can be attributed not only to the design of the diffractive lens array, delivering high-energy microbeams, but also to the optical of absorption of melanin to 755 nm wavelength delivered at sub-nanosecond pulses. The inherent absorption of the alexandrite wavelength by melanin is greater than that of hemoglobin allowing for the production of LIOB without hemorrhage as seen with 1064 nm and 532 nm.[27]

To validate the safety and efficacy of "picotoning" on darker skin types, Tanghetti and Shin evaluated 20 Asian patients with Fitzpatrick skin types IV and V receiving 3 to 5 treatments every 2 to 4 weeks with an 8 mm (0.40 j/cm$^2$) FOCUS lens. Patients received between 5000 and 6000 pulses delivered over 3 to 4 passes. Posttreatment results indicated a 90% to 95% reduction in pigmentation, 70% to 75% improvement in texture, and 50% to 60% improvement in pore size.[28]

The authors, in their clinic, recommend using the 8- or 10-mm flat or FOCUS lens in darker skin type individuals, with long duration intervals between treatments (4–6 weeks) to allow for healing and visualization of any issues with pigmentation. Pulse counts between 3000 and 5000 are often used, and areas are treated per quadrant until mild, confluent erythema is noted.

## OFF-FACE APPLICATIONS

Laser toning, before PicoSure, has primarily been for facial photodamage. The exact mechanism of laser toning is not thoroughly known; however, it has been proposed that melanin granules are fragmented and dispersed into the cytoplasm without cellular destruction by repetitive laser energy with a sub-photothermolytic fluence delivery.[29]

Although minimization of pigmentation does occur, the longer pulse durations were not substantive to induce thermal or acoustic dermal remodeling to affect textural irregularities of the face. Off-the-body applications are challenging as less dermal adnexal structures are present for healing and dyspigmentation, and textural irregularity can result.

Picotoning lends itself to off-body applications with the use of FOCUS lens. Several initial studies were performed on the décolletage[30,31] and the dorsum of the hands[31] with documented improvements in rhytid reduction and pigmentation (**Figs. 10** and **11**). Although topical numbing is helpful in the décolletage area, it is not necessary for the dorsum of the hands.

Other off-face applications include treatment of hemosiderin staining in patients postsclerotherapy. One to two treatments with the 6-mm FOCUS lens are recommended to minimize the pigmentary alteration (**Fig. 12**).

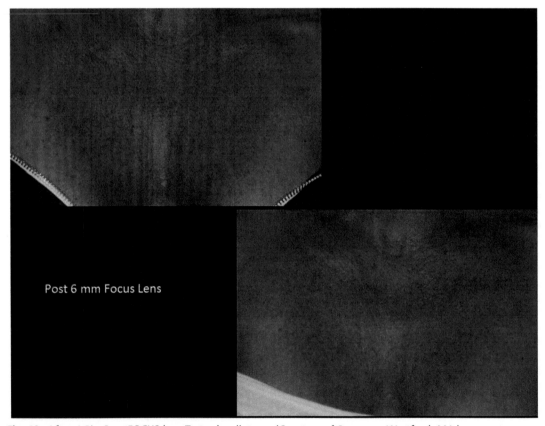

Post 6 mm Focus Lens

**Fig. 10.** After 4 PicoSure FOCUS lens Tx to decolletage. (*Courtesy of* Cynosure, Westford, MA.)

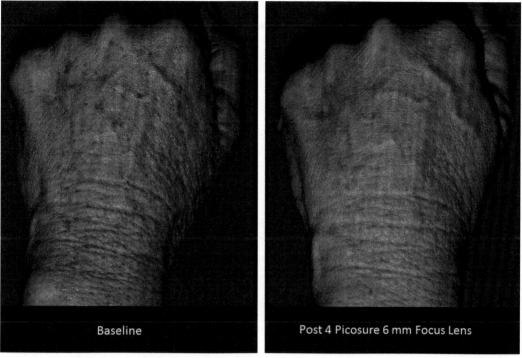

Baseline

Post 4 Picosure 6 mm Focus Lens

**Fig. 11.** After 4 PicoSure FOCUS lens Tx to dorsum of hand with improvement of texture and pigmentation. (*Courtesy of* Cynosure, Westford, MA.)

## MELASMA

Melasma is one of the most challenging cutaneous issues to treat. Before any treatment, it is recommended for the skin to be "primed" with topical retinoic acid, a bleaching agent, and a photoprotector such as topical vitamin C/E/Ferulic serum. Patients should practice strict sun protection with a tinted (iron oxide), physical blocking sunscreen (zinc and titanium), as visible light as well as ultraviolet radiation can worsen melasma. Mandatory evaluation posttreatment is required, as a percentage of patients with melasma can worsen with laser irradiation.

With multiple modalities of lasers available, the authors opt for a low-level treatment starting either with an 8 or 10 mm flat lens in Fitz IV and higher and 6-mm FOCUS in Fitzpatrick skin types 3 and lower. The authors typically treat with a 5 Hz repetition rate (or lower) and deliver between 1500 and 3500 pulses until the melasma darkens. Treatments are performed every 6 weeks to evaluate for any postinflammatory hyperpigmentation. With this conservative method, improvement can be visualized in most of the patients in whom laser may be an option (**Figs. 13** and **14**). If any darkening occurs after 2 treatments, laser treatment is aborted and continued with topicals. Prelaser discussions regarding periodic maintenance is important to communicate.

## MULTIPLE-WAVELENGTH PICO LASERS
### Discovery Pico Plus

Discovery Pico Plus™ (**Fig. 15**) (Quanta System S.p.A, Milan, Italy), an FDA-approved second-generation picosecond laser, uses Quanta's patented Pico-Boost technology to generate the highest peak power among available picosecond lasers such as PicoSure, Picoway, Lutronic Pico-Plus, Enlighten, etc. Multiple-wavelength Pico lasers haveblossomed since 2014, with most adopting the 1064/532 frequency-doubled platform including the Picoway, Pico Plus, Enlighten, and PiQ04, some of which use handpiece configurations to obtain multi-wavelength capabilities (**Fig. 16**). Discovery Pico Plus has 1.8 GW peak power, which is many times higher than regular nanosecond Q-switched lasers such as the Fotona StarWalker MaQX (which has a 5-ns pulse duration and is not a picosecond laser) that have peak powers ranging from 0.2 to 0.5 GW. Higher peak power laser pulses can break up pigments more thoroughly and at a deeper depth in the

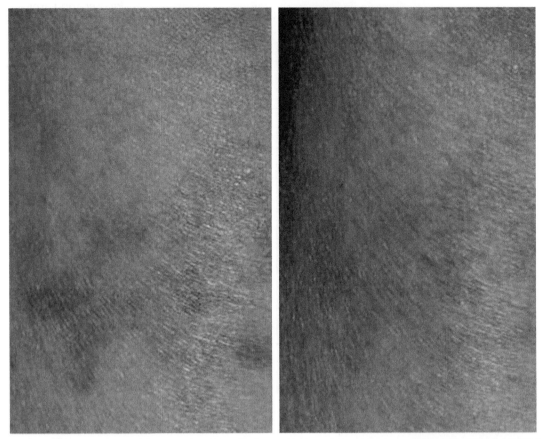

**Fig. 12.** After 1 treatment with 6-mm FOCUS lens for hemosiderin staining. (*Courtesy of* Cynosure, Westford, MA.)

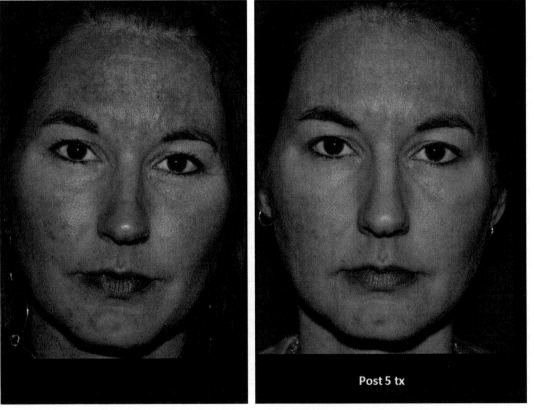

Post 5 tx

**Fig. 13.** After 5 FOCUS lens, 6 mm Tx for melasma. (*Courtesy of* Cynosure, Westford, MA.)

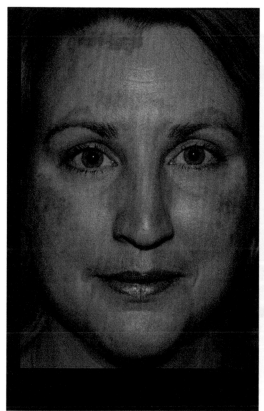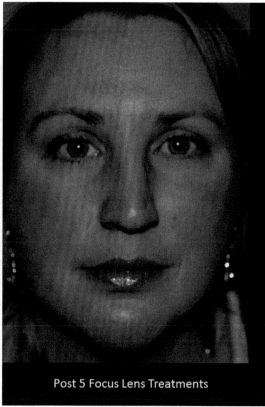

Post 5 Focus Lens Treatments

**Fig. 14.** After 5 PicoSure FOCUS lens Tx with 6 mm for melasma. (*Courtesy of* Cynosure, Westford, MA.)

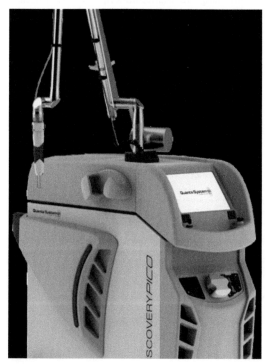

**Fig. 15.** Quanta discovery Pico Plus. (*Courtesy of* Quanta System, Samarate, Italy; with permission.)

skin, making it more effective for stubborn pigmentation.

### Triple-Wavelength with Full-Powered Ruby Wavelength

Green (frequency-doubled Nd:YAG—532 nm), red (ruby—694 nm), and infrared (Nd:YAG—1064 nm) laser light can be emitted. Quanta Discovery Pico Plus houses a full-powered ruby laser. Other q-switched picosecond or nanosecond lasers use dye convertor handpieces requiring a 2-step wavelength conversion with high conversion losses, leading to inadequate power and hence slower and less effective treatments. For example, a full-powered nanosecond NdYAG laser with 1600 mJ energy per pulse would only be able to produce a 220 mJ pulse after conversion, compared with the 1200 mJ of the Quanta Discovery Pico Plus. A third wavelength with adequate power is essential for treating notoriously difficult to eradicate green, sky blue, and blue tattoos effectively. The higher melanin absorption of the ruby wavelength also makes it more effective for clearing pigmentation without producing complications

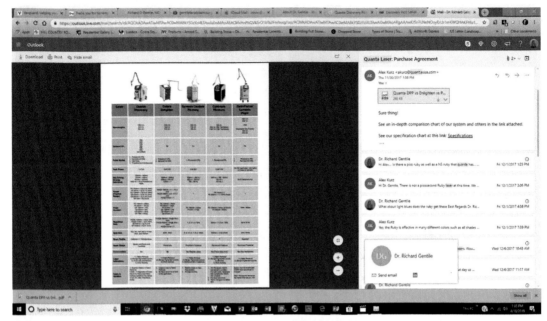

**Fig. 16.** Pico laser summary sheet. (*Courtesy of* Cynosure, Westford, MA; with permission.)

such as postinflammatory hyperpigmentation or blistering.

### Adjustable Pulse Duration with Four Emission Modes

Unlike many other picosecond lasers that can only produce picosecond pulses, Quanta Discovery Pico Plus is able to produce picosecond, nanosecond, OptiPulse (double nanosecond) to quasi-long pulsed 300 us pulse durations. This adjustable pulse duration allows the physician to customize the desired effect of the laser, using ultrashort pulse durations for photoacoustic effects (for breaking up pigmentation, scar treatments) and longer ones for photothermal effects (to treat acne, stimulate collagen production).

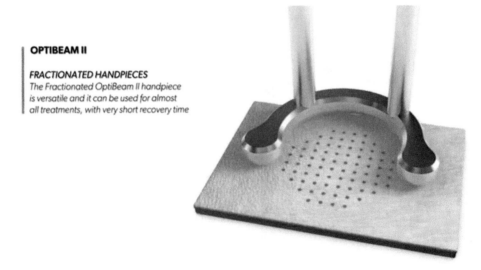

**Fig. 17.** Fractionated OptiBeam II handpiece. The Fractionated OptiBeam II handpiece is versatile and it can be used for almost all treatments, with very short recovery time. (*Courtesy of* Quanta System, Samarate, Italy; with permission.)

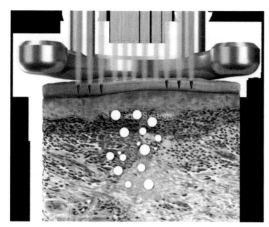

**Fig. 18.** Multilevel LIOB.

## Fractional Microlens Array

Quanta Discovery Pico Plus laser uses a special fractional microlens array (MLA) handpiece to further concentrate the laser energy into tiny spots (**Fig. 17**). These areas of extremely high energy can generate LIOB leading to plasma formation, cavitation, and shockwave formation. This effectively breaks down scar tissue and old collagen and activates intense collagen stimulation leading to skin renewal, improvement in skin texture, scarring, and pore size.

## Multilevel Picosecond Effect

Discovery PICO's fractional treatments take advantage of 2 different laser actions with the creation of LIOBs for collagen remodeling and the ablation of damaged skin through picosecond "cold" ablation. The synergy between these 2 effects is the key to the success in full treatment of wrinkles and acne scars (**Fig. 18**).

## Twain Handpieces for Discovery Pico Plus

Optional Twain options are IPL or Er:YAG handpieces that can be attached to the Twain connector of the device. Twain IPL is indicated for permanent hair reduction, dermatologic vascular lesions, benign pigmented lesions, and inflammatory acne. Twain 2940 is indicated for skin resurfacing, treatment of wrinkles, epidermal nevi, actinis cheilitis, keloids, verrucae, skin tags, keratoses, scar revision (including acne scars), and with microbeam handpiece it is indicated for skin resurfacing.

## SUMMARY

PicoSure and pico pulsed lasers with the zoom handpiece and flat and FOCUS lens and other versions of MLA have contributed to our ability to safely treat tattoo ink, benign pigmentation, rhytides, scarring, and striae in both lighter and darker Fitzpatrick skin type individuals.

## DISCLOSURES

None.

## REFERENCES

1. Einstein A. 1925.Quantentheorie des einatomigen idealen Gases, Zweite Abhandlung Sitz. Preussischen Akad. Wiss. 8 3.
2. Qian P, Juzeniene A, Chen J, et al. Lasers in medicine. Rep Prog Phys 2008;71. 056701 (28pp).
3. Anderson RR, Parrish JA. Selective photothermolysis: precise microsurgery by selective absorption of pulsed radiation. Science 1983;220(4596):524–7.
4. Ross V, Naseef G, Lin G, et al. Comparison of responses of tattoos to picosecond and nanosecond Q-switched neodymium:YAG lasers. Arch Dermatol 1998;134:167–71.
5. Herd RM, Alora MB, Smoller B, et al. A clinical and histologic prospective controlled comparative study of the picosecond titanium:sapphire (795 nm) laser versus the Q-switched alexandrite (752 nm) laser for removing tattoo pigment. J Am Acad Dermatol 1999;40(4):603–6.
6. Ho DD, London R, Zimmerman GB, et al. Laser-tattoo removal–a study of the mechanism and the optimal treatment strategy via computer simulations. Lasers Surg Med 2002;30(5):389–97.
7. Mirkov M, Sierra R. Impact of pulse duration from nanoseconds to picoseconds on the thermal and mechanical effects during the laser interaction with tattoo targets. ASLMS podium presentation. Boston, Massachusetts, April 3–7, 2013.
8. Paltauf G, Dyer PE. Photomechanical processes and effects in ablation. Chem Rev 2003;103(2):487–518.
9. Kazandjieva J, Tsankov N. Tattoos: dermatological complications. Clin Dermatol 2007;25:375–82.
10. Brauer JA, Reddy KK, Anolik R, et al. Successful and rapid treatment of blue and green tattoo pigment with a novel picosecond laser. Arch Dermatol 2012;148(7):820–3.
11. Saedi N, Metelitsa A, Petrell K, et al. Treatment of tattoos with a picosecond alexandrite laser: a prospective trial. Arch Dermatol 2012;148(12):1360–3.
12. Gomez C, Martin V, Sastre R, et al. In vitro and in vivo laser treatments of tattoos: high efficiency and low fluences. Arch Dermatol 2010;146(1):39–45.
13. Beute TC, Miller CH, Timko AL, et al. In vitro spectral analysis of tattoo pigments. Dermatol Surg 2008; 34(4):508–15 [discussion: 515–6].
14. Alabdulrazzaq H, Brauer JA, Bae YS, et al. Clearance of yellow tattoo ink with a novel 532- nm picosecond laser. Lasers Surg Med 2015;47:285–8.

15. Gusev VE, Karabutov AA. Lazernaya Optoakuslika (Naoka, Moscow, 1991). [Laser Optoacoustics]. New York: AIP Press; 1993.

16. Izikson L, Farinelli W, Sakamoto F, et al. Safety and effectiveness of blacktattoo clearance in a pig model after a single treatment with a novel 758nm 500 picosecond laser: a pilot study. Lasers Surg Med 2010;42(7):640–6.

17. Kirby W, Desai A, Desai T, et al. The Kirby-Desai scale. A proposed scale to assess tattoo-removal treatment. J Clin Aesthet Dermatol 2009;2(3):32–7.

18. Tanghetti EA. The histology of skin treated with a picosecond alexandrite laser and a fractional lens array. Lasers Surg Med 2016. https://doi.org/10.1002/lsm.22540.

19. Rockwell BA, Thomas RJ, Vogel A, et al. Ultrashort laser pulse retinal damage mechanisms and their impact on thresholds. Med Laser Appl 2010;25: 84–92.

20. Uzunbajakava N, Varghese B, Botchkareva V, et al. Highlighting the nuances behind interaction of picosecond pulses with human skin: relating distinct laser-tissue interactions to their potential in cutaneous intervensions. San Francisco (CA): SPIE BiOS; 2018.

21. McDaniel D. Gene expression analysis in cultured human skin fibroblasts following exposure to a Picosecond Pulsed Alexandrite laser and specially designed focus optic. Lasers Surg Med 2015; 47(S26):22.

22. Brauer JA, Kazlouskaya V, Alabdulrazzaq H, et al. Use of a picosecond pulse duration laser with specialized optic for treatment of facial acne scarring. JAMA Dermatol 2015;151(3):278–84.

23. Tanghettii E, Tartar DM. Comparison of the cutaneous thermal signatures over twenty-four hours with a picosecond alexandrite laser using a flat or fractional optic. J Drugs Dermatol 2016;15(11): 1347–52.

24. Dierickx C. Using normal and high pulse coverage with picosecond laser treatment of wrinkles and acne scarring: long term clinical observation. Lasers Surg Med 2018;50:51–5.

25. Weiss R, McDaniel DH, Weiss MA, et al. Safety and efficacy of a novel diffractive lens array using a picosecond 755 nm Alexandrite laser for treatment of wrinkles. Lasers Surg Med 2017;49: 40–4.

26. Chan NP, Ho SG, Shek SY, et al. A case series of facial depigmentation associated with low fluence Q-switched 1,064nm Nd:YAG laser for skin rejuvenation and melasma. Lasers Surg Med 2010;42:712.

27. Lee MC, Hu S, Chen MC, et al. Skin rejuvenation with 1,064-nm Q-switched Nd:YAG laser in Asian patients. Dermatol Surg 2009;35:929–32.

28. Shin, Tanghetti. Picotoning: a Novel laser toning approach for the treatment of Asian skin types. White Paper.

29. Mun JY, Jeong SY, Kim JH, et al. A low fluence Q-switched Nd:YAG laser modifies the 3D structure of melanocyte and ultrastructure of melanosome by subcellular-selective photothermoloysis. J Electron Microsc (Tokyo) 2011;60:11–8.

30. Wu DC, Fletcher L, Guiha I, et al. Evaluation of the safety and efficacy of the picosecond alexandrite laser with specializedlens array for treatment of the photoagingdecolletage. Lasers Surg Med 2016; 48(2):188–92.

31. Saluja R. Evaluation of the safety and efficacy of a low fluence, picopulsed, alexandrite laser in a pico-toning technique with a diffractive lens optic for the treatment of photodamage and textural improvement in "off the face" application. J Drugs Dermatol 2016;15(11).

# New Frontiers in Skin Rejuvenation, Including Stem Cells and Autologous Therapies

Aunna Pourang, MD[a], Helena Rockwell, BSc[b], Kian Karimi, MD[c],*

## KEYWORDS

- Stem cells • Rejuvenation • Aesthetic • Cosmetic • Fat transfer • Platelet therapy • Adipose
- Thread lift

## KEY POINTS

- Minimally invasive cosmetic procedures are increasing in demand and popularity with a recent trend toward a more natural look.
- Autologous therapies, such as adipose-derived stem cells, stromal vascular fraction, microfat, nanofat, and platelet therapies, have been shown to effectively rejuvenate the skin.
- Innovations in botulinum toxin, fillers, and thread lifts parallel the increasing trends in autologous therapy use in aesthetic medicine.
- A combination approach using both autologous and traditional aesthetic therapies can provide optimal aesthetic outcomes.

 Video content accompanies this article at http://www.facialplastic.theclinics.com.

## INTRODUCTION

Minimally invasive cosmetic procedures continue to dominate the aesthetic arena. There are a large number of younger patients requesting cosmetic procedures with a focus on maintaining a youthful, natural look.[1] For this reason, so-called prejuvenation has become a popular aesthetic goal for many.

There is nothing more natural than a person's own tissues. Autologous therapies are increasingly being implemented for skin rejuvenation purposes in individuals of all ages. Using an individual's own fat, yielding nanofat, adipose-derived stem cells (ASCs), and stromal vascular fraction, as well as

platelets and fibrin from the person's blood, aging can be delayed or "reversed" with relative safety and efficacy. Much of the research on autologous therapy is in its infancy, but this revolutionary technology holds great promise.

Noninvasive cosmetic procedures, in general, continue to dominate aesthetics. New developments in technologies of botulinum toxin, fillers, and threads provide patients with multiple options. A combination approach of all available interventions can be used in clinical practice to provide patients with optimal, tailored skin rejuvenation.

Disclosure: K. Karimi is the medical director of CosmoFrance, Inc, which manufactures and distributes platelet-rich fibrin centrifuges and tubes as well as polydioxanone (PDO) threads. A. Pourang has served as a faculty member for LearnSkin.com. H. Rockwell has no relevant financial disclosures.

[a] Department of Dermatology, University of California, Davis, 3301 C Street, Suite 1400, Sacramento, CA 95816, USA; [b] University of California, San Diego, School of Medicine, 9500 Gilman Drive, La Jolla, CA 92093, USA; [c] Rejuva Medical Aesthetics, 11645 Wilshire Boulevard #605, Los Angeles, CA 90025, USA
* Corresponding author.
*E-mail address:* kiankarimi@gmail.com

Facial Plast Surg Clin N Am 28 (2020) 101–117
https://doi.org/10.1016/j.fsc.2019.09.009
1064-7406/20/© 2019 Elsevier Inc. All rights reserved.

## Regenerative Medicine

The therapeutic potential for autologous therapy is an area of medicine that continues to be explored in many fields, from orthopedics to dermatology and plastic surgery.[2] An individual's tissues and cells are processed outside of the body and reintroduced back into the donor, with minimal risk of hypersensitivity reactions. Autologous therapies vary and involve different cell types and growth factors that help regenerate tissues.

## Stem Cells

The regenerative potential of stem cells has expanded beyond the treatment of chronic degenerative diseases and into aesthetic medicine. Compared with embryonic stem cells or induced pluripotent stem cells, mesenchymal stem cells (MSCs) are preferred for use in clinical practice given the high availability, ability to differentiate into many cell types, and relative lack of ethical concerns.[2]

ASCs are the multipotent MSC population found in the stromal vascular fraction (SVF) of fat tissue, with the ability to differentiate into mesoderm, ectoderm, and endoderm lineages.[3–5] ASCs also show regenerative and wound healing properties.[6,7] They can be obtained from adipose tissue in large quantities using a standard wet liposuction procedure under local anesthesia, with minimal discomfort and morbidity of the patient, and without the need for expansion in culture, in contrast with bone marrow MSCs (BM-MSCs).[8,9] Other sources of stem cells include amniotic fluid stem cells, umbilical cord blood stem cells, and Wharton jelly, which have greater proliferative and differentiation potential compared with ASCs and BM-MSCs, but are limited in cell availability after in vitro expansion.[10–12]

Different methods of ASC isolation have been described in the literature.[2,13–15] Lipoaspirate is harvested by using tumescent abdominal liposuction techniques or surgical resection.[16] ASCs are usually isolated by collagenase digestion of isolated white adipose tissue, followed by centrifugation to separate the SVF-containing ASCs in the pellet fraction from floating adipocytes and blood.[8,17–19] SVF is the heterogeneous mixture of cells obtained by enzymatic separation of adipocytes, and contains fibroblasts, endothelial cells, monocytes, macrophages, granulocytes, and lymphocytes.[20,21]

ASCs can ultimately be isolated from SVF after separation from adipocytes and can be cultured to form fibroblast-like colonies.[20] ASCs used alone after expansion in vitro or with SVF are the most common MSCs used in aesthetic dermatology and plastic surgery practice.[2] Because pure ASCs alone require in vitro expansion, which can be time consuming and labor intensive, SVF is often used because it already contains ASCs.

### Mechanisms of action and clinical applications

The regenerative potential of SVF and ASCs is thought to be caused by various mechanisms. The regenerative ability of the skin is maintained by the stem cells that are present in the hair follicle, interfollicular epidermis, and sebaceous glands, as well as being influenced by mesenchymal-epithelial crosstalk through secreted stimulatory factors.[22–25] Intradermal adipocyte lineage cells have been found to be necessary in driving hair follicle stem cell activation and likely play a role in other epithelial stem cell functions.[24,26] ASCs are also thought to stimulate the recruitment of endogenous stem cells and promote their differentiation to cells that are needed, such as at a site of tissue injury.[13] In addition, stem cells, in general, have antioxidant capabilities that likely mitigate inflammation and wound healing.[27] Some investigators suggest that the preadipocytes and macrophages in SVF confer regenerative properties through enhanced immune response or removal of dying cells, leading to tissue remodeling.[28,29] Both SVF and ASCs are thought to have properties that increase vascularization, the secretion of growth factors, vascular endothelial growth factor (VEGF), hepatocyte growth factor, and insulinlike growth factor.[30–34] Such properties are also likely responsible for enhancing fat graft survival.

Cultured ASCs have been shown to improve scar outcomes of full-thickness skin defects.[35] Cultured ASCs have also been found to reduce wrinkles through collagen and elastic fiber production and other antiaging effects in the skin through glycation suppression, antioxidation, and trophic effects.[36,37] SVF, which contains ASCs, has also been used to treat necrosis resulting from facial filler injections.[38,39]

### Scientific evidence and regulatory issues

It is important to keep in mind that stem cell technology is still in its infancy, with US Food and Drug Administration (FDA)–approved trials in early phases.[2,24,40] Potential side effects of stem cells such as rejection, hyperimmune response, neoplasm, cross contamination with other stem cell lines, and uncontrolled differentiation have been proposed.[41–44] Human ASCs that have been cultured in vitro for long periods of time have been found to produce tumors in immunodeficient mice.[45] There is also a question as to whether or not the donor's age affects the regenerative potential of ASCs.[46] The lack of safety and potential side effects data are limited and further randomized clinical trials are necessary.[2] Furthermore, there is no single standard protocol for obtaining ASCs, which can lead to regulatory and quality issues.[6,47]

Some clinicians are even calling on the FDA to expedite the oversight of companies and clinics offering stem cell–based treatments.[48] Procedures are being offered in some spalike settings and are at risk for contamination and infection. Professional groups are requesting that stem cell products be regulated like drugs, that the scope of practice for such procedures be regulated, and that these procedures be performed in state or national facilities accredited by surgical associations.

## Fat Transfer

Fat transfer procedures (**Table 1**) are becoming increasingly popular given it is a relatively safe autologous therapy, helping reverse volume loss with the added benefit of removing unwanted fat. Lipofilling procedures are often used to correct dark circles and hollows around the eyes, volumize the midface, and augment the chin[20,49–51] (**Fig. 1**). Adipose tissue is not only an ideal filler because of its ability to integrate into a donor's tissues with minimal risk of immunogenicity but also contains several cell types with regenerative potential, as discussed earlier, which can rejuvenate the skin of the face.[52–54] The ASCs in the fat have been shown to promote new collagen deposition, local hypervascularity, and dermal hyperplasia.[55,56]

### Microfat, superficial enhanced fluid fat injection, and nanofat

Successful fat grafting depends on several factors, including proper procedural technique, the possibility of needing multiple treatments, and optimization of the recipient site's capacity to support the graft.[59] Disadvantages of traditional fat grafting, which uses large blunt cannulas, include the risks of irregular fat accumulation, visible lumpiness, fat necrosis, and poor fat graft survival.[20,60]

Mechanical and enzymatic disruption of fat has been shown to improve the viability of adipocytes and graft retention.[20,61–63] Microfat is generated by using a smaller multiport cannula, as small as 0.7 mm in diameter, and is then injected intradermally to treat fine wrinkles.[64–66] Superficial enhanced fluid fat injection (SEFFI) is a procedure that was developed to overcome manual centrifugation's effects on adipocyte viability.[57] Micro side-port cannulae are used to harvest microfat rich in stem cells and viable adipocytes, which is then enhanced with autologous platelet-rich plasma (PRP) and injected

superficially with syringe needles. This treatment has been shown to result in lump-free skin rejuvenation and volume enhancement.[58] Micro-SEFFI (M-SEFFI) is a refined version of the SEFFI procedure, obtaining smoother fat, harvested with a multiperforated cannula with extremely small ports (0.3 mm).[21]

Nanofat is generated by further processing of fat via mechanical emulsification. Tonnard and colleagues[20] describe their procedure for nanofat production in which standard high-negative-pressure liposuction is used to harvest fat using a multiport 3-mm cannula with sharp side holes of 1 mm in diameter. After saline rinsing and filtering, adipose tissue is then emulsified by shifting the fat 30 times between two 10-mL syringes connected by a female-to-female Luer-Lok connector to create an emulsion, which is filtered over a sterile nylon cloth. The remaining effluent without connective tissue is called nanofat, yielding 1 mL of nanofat per 10 mL of lipoaspirate (Video 1). Nanofat is layered fanwise intradermally using a 27-gauge needle in delicate areas such as superficial rhytids and eyelids, with a delayed effect usually appearing within 4 weeks to 3 months. Nanofat does not contain viable adipocytes, limiting its ability to volumize tissue, but retains high levels of ASCs, which can be used for skin rejuvenation purposes. It is thought that increased collagen and elastin formation and skin remodeling occurs because of the ASCs.[20]

Nanofat injection may be a less expensive, less time-consuming way of introducing beneficial stem cells to surrounding tissues, because SVF would need to be further isolated from the nanofat's dead adipocyte fraction.[20] The fragmented adipocyte portion may even be beneficial because it can induce cytokine release and growth factors, which can help regenerate tissue.[20,67]

### Combination therapies

ASCs from processed adipose tissue are often combined with macrofat grafts to improve outcomes. Although nanofat alone is typically used for skin rejuvenation, it is often combined with macrofat grafts. Gu and colleagues[68] used condensed nanofat, removing oil that was thought to be too bulky to inject into scars, combined with fat grafts to effectively treat atrophic facial scars.

Cell-assisted lipotransfer (CAL), a technique in which fat grafts are enriched with SVF, has been shown to improve fat transfer in facial lipoatrophy compared with conventional lipoinjection, along with a decreased risk of fibrosis, pseudocyst formation, and calcification as seen with traditional lipoinjection.[69,70]

**Table 1**
**Types of autologous fat therapy**

| Cell Type | Mechanism of Extraction | Pros | Cons | Contain Viable Adipocytes? | Contains ASCs? |
|---|---|---|---|---|---|
| Macrofat | Standard liposuction using large multiport cannula | Good filler | Granuloma formation<br>Lumps<br>Fat necrosis<br>Calcification<br>Poor graft retention possible<br>May need multiple treatments | Yes | Yes |
| Microfat | Liposuction using small multiport cannula | Good filler<br>Rejuvenates skin | Same as macrofat | Yes | Yes |
| SEFFI[57] | Liposuction using small multiport cannula (0.8 and 0.5 mm) + PRP | Finer than microfat<br>Good filler<br>Rejuvenates skin<br>Does not require further tissue manipulation<br>Includes PRP growth factors | Oil cyst formation reported in some patients<br>Requires additional procedure (PRP) | Yes | Yes |
| M-SEFFI[58] | Liposuction using small multiport cannula (0.3 mm) + PRP | Finer than SEFFI<br>Good filler<br>Rejuvenates skin<br>Does not require further tissue manipulation<br>Includes PRP growth factors | Requires additional procedure (PRP) | Yes | Yes |
| Nanofat[20] | Liposuction using multiport 3-mm cannula with sharp side holes of 1 mm in diameter with subsequent emulsification of microfat, filtered to remove connective tissue | Rejuvenates skin | Suboptimal filler<br>Requires additional processing after liposuction | No | Yes |
| SVF[2] | Lipoaspirate undergoes processing using enzymatic or mechanical separation and is then washed, treated with collagenase, centrifuged, and red blood cells are removed | Inexpensive<br>Applied during 1 surgical procedure | Not purely ASCs (heterogeneous cell fraction), which is still beneficial<br>Requires additional processing after liposuction | No | Yes |
| ASC (alone, after expansion in vitro)[2] | Culture from SVF | Obtain homogeneous cell fraction with fully defined phenotype | Cost and time intensive<br>Potential tumorigenic ability<br>Requires additional processing and culturing after liposuction | No | Yes |

*Abbreviations:* PRP, platelet-rich plasma; M-SEFFI, micro–superficial enhanced fluid fat injection; SEFFI, superficial enhanced fluid fat injection.

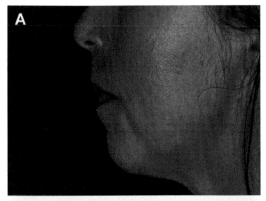

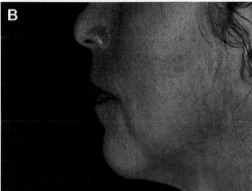

**Fig. 1.** (*A*) Before and (*B*) after chin augmentation with autologous microfat graft purifed by PureGraft (Bimini Technologies, Solana Beach, CA) mixed with autologous PRF obtained using ezPRF System.

## Autologous Platelet Therapies

Despite origins in oral maxillofacial surgery,[71,72] autologous platelet therapies have been found to be useful in several other clinical fields, including aesthetics. This usefulness is largely caused by the existence of parallels between the body's innate mechanisms of wound healing, in which platelets play a major contributing role, and the pathways necessary for rejuvenation. First, there was platelet-rich plasma (PRP)[71,72] but, with the turn of the century, came the emergence of platelet-rich fibrin (PRF).[73]

### Mechanism of action

As cellular constituents of whole blood, platelets are among the first responders to sites of tissue and vascular injury. In such events, platelet aggregation and activation result in the release of several critical growth factors from platelet alpha granules, including platelet-derived growth factor, fibroblastic growth factor, epithelial growth factor, insulinlike growth factor,

transforming growth factor, and VEGF,[74–77] which are further described in **Table 2**.

The chemotactic properties of these growth factors serve, in part, to recruit MSCs, which then differentiate at the site of injury.[77–79] Furthermore, during this process of response to injury, the enzyme thrombin converts the soluble blood protein fibrinogen into insoluble fibrin. Fibrin then acts as a binding scaffold for erythrocytes and platelets to stabilize clot formation, establishing a fibrin matrix for subsequent remodeling, and sustaining growth factors.[77,80–83] It is these growth

| Table 2<br>Growth factors found in platelet therapies and their functions | |
|---|---|
| **Growth Factor** | **Functions** |
| PDGF | • Stimulates fibroblasts and leukocytes such as neutrophils and macrophages<br>• Chemotactically recruits MSCs, endothelial cells, and fibroblasts, and stimulates their replication<br>• Important for blood vessel maturation<br>• Collagen production |
| FGF | • Mitogenic for fibroblasts and endothelial cells<br>• Facilitates repair of soft tissues<br>• Angiogenic effects lay groundwork for the synthesis, deposition, organization, and ultimate formation of extracellular matrix<br>• Hyaluronic acid production<br>• Collagenesis |
| EGF | • Regulates proliferation, growth, and the migration of epithelial cells<br>• Angiogenic |
| IGF | • Promotes cell growth |
| TGFβ | • Mitogenic and morphogenic functions<br>• Promotes wound healing<br>• The TGFβ3 isoform inhibits haphazard scarring and promotes cellular differentiation and replication<br>• Stimulates collagenesis |
| VEGF | • Angiogenic<br>• Facilitates extracellular matrix synthesis and deposition |

*Abbreviations:* EGF, epithelial growth factor; FGF, fibroblastic growth factor; IGF, insulinlike growth factor; PDGF, platelet-derived growth factor; TGFβ, transforming growth factor beta.

factors that ultimately orchestrate the healing, regenerative, and rejuvenating properties of platelets. Thus, by using blood concentrates such as PRP and PRF, clinicians can selectively implement the clinically relevant effects of platelet growth factors.

### Platelet-rich plasma and platelet-rich fibrin

PRP and PRF are acquired by centrifuging whole blood for product-specific durations of time and either with or without additives (**Fig. 2**). PRP and PRF primarily differ in their respective preparation, rate of growth factor release, and mode of activation for clot formation. These basic differences and similarities and several others are summarized in **Table 3**.

### Platelet-rich plasma versus platelet-rich fibrin

The preferred use of PRF compared with PRP is well justified. First, without the need for additives, as is the case with PRP, preparation and use of PRF confers reduced costs for patients and providers as well as a more standardized protocol that is less susceptible to human error. Furthermore, PRF is a completely autologous product, whereas PRP, as a result of its preparation, is not; thus, PRP presents the risk of inducing an adverse immune response.[88]

With continued consideration of their differences in preparation, the high-speed versus low-speed centrifugation parameters of PRP and PRF preparation, respectively, diversify their composition. As a result of low-speed centrifugation, a greater proportion of the beneficial cellular content of blood is preserved within the resulting PRF layer,[84,91] whereas the high-speed centrifugation of PRP pushes many cells toward the hematocrit,[86,91] which is ultimately unused and discarded.

PRF further surpasses PRP with regard to growth factor release. The rapid activation and release of growth factors in PRP has been noted to yield short-term benefits without long-term advances in wound healing.[90] Contrastingly, the natural, physiologic activation of PRF and its prolonged growth factor release sustains healing and regenerative signals for a longer period of time.[90] In addition, in 1 particular study, PRF was found to yield higher overall concentrations of growth factors than PRP.[92]

Although the growth factor signaling of both PRP and PRF attracts MSC migration to sites of implementation and injury, PRF has been shown to contain multipotent stem cell markers and carry cells that bear phenotypic features that are characteristic of MSCs.[93] As a result, PRF serves not only to attract and sustain MSCs with its autologous and naturally forming fibrin matrix but may also serve as a reservoir of these regenerative and rejuvenating cells.

Collectively, these findings, as well as other comparative studies and reviews documented in the literature, support PRF's superiority to PRP for use as a wound healing and regenerative aid.[86,94–96]

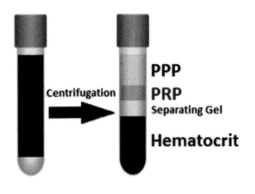
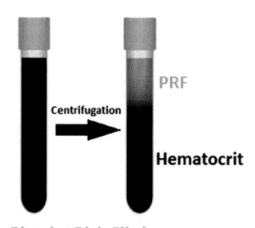

**Fig. 2.** The generation of PRP from whole blood (*left*) and PRF from whole blood (*right*) from centrifugation. The supernatant contains the desired product, whereas the hematocrit, consisting of concentrated red blood cells, constitutes the inferior subsection of the solution, and is discarded. PPP, platelet-poor plasma. (*Courtesy of* CosmoFrance Inc., Miami, Florida and *modified from* Karimi K, Rockwell H. The Benefits of Platelet Rich Fibrin (PRF). Facial Plastic Surgery Clinics. 2019;27(3); with permission.)

| | PRP | PRF |
|---|---|---|
| ...n | Generally higher speeds | Generally lower speeds |
| | Whole blood is spun with anticoagulant and separating gel | Whole blood is spun without any additives |
| Activation ... coagulation (Fibrin P... rization/Clot Formatio... -89 | Induced by the addition of thrombin (often bovine derived) and calcium chloride or entrusted to be stimulated by endogenous coagulation factors after application/injection | Spontaneous; natural cascade of coagulation and fibrin clot formation based on intrinsic processes |
| Growth Factor Release Rate[85,90] | Rapid release of growth factors on implementation (~24 h) | Prolonged duration of growth factor release (~7–10 d) |
| Leukocyte Content[86,87] | 0%–50% of cells in supernatant product; lower retention | ~65% of cells in supernatant product; higher retention |
| MSC Recruitment[77,87] | Chemotactically attracts MSC migration | Chemotactically attracts MSC migration |
| Lifespan of Fibrin Matrix Clot After Application[86] | Dissolves quickly after application | Processed slowly; gradually, physiologically remodeled |

## APPLICATIONS OF PLATELET-RICH PLASMA AND PLATELET-RICH FIBRIN

PRP and PRF boast an array of surgical and nonsurgical aesthetic applications, including improved retention of fat grafts, hair restoration, optimizing cartilage grafts in rhinoplasty, improving scar appearance, collagen induction therapy, ablative laser resurfacing, and volumization both independently and in conjunction with hyaluronic acid filler.[97,98]

### Implications as an Injectable

As people age, the collagen, elastin, subcutaneous fat, and hyaluronic acid content of the facial skin declines,[99] which manifests as facial hollowness, drooping skin, and the formation of rhytids. It has been suggested that injection of growth factors stimulates dermal collagen synthesis.[75] PRP's target site–specific growth factor release has been shown to promote fibroblast proliferation and stimulate both type I collagenesis[100] and hyaluronic acid production.[98] Although PRP is known to enhance the duration of the effects from hyaluronic acid filler treatments,[98] the prolonged release of growth factors[85] and physiologic rate of remodeling of the PRF fibrin matrix[86] is hypothesized to further improve the duration of hyaluronic acid filler

treatments. Author K.K. has observed this effect in his own practice with patients who have received both treatment with filler alone as well as filler combined with PRF for injection. Injecting PRF provides an immediate volumization effect that diminishes over the following few weeks; however, anecdotal evidence from repeat treatments of PRF by author K.K. has suggested long-term improvements in facial volume, skin texture, and skin pigmentation when used as a lone autologous dermal filler (**Fig. 3**).[97]

### Microneedling

Microneedling, or collagen induction therapy, is a popular, minimal-downtime procedure known to improve skin texture, the presence of fine lines and scars, and enhance skin appearance without risks of hyperpigmentation.[101] This superficial, controlled puncturing of the skin by very fine needles stimulates the wound healing response, ultimately leading to the release of growth factors by platelets and neocollagenesis. Topical application of growth factors has been shown to improve skin texture and appearance[102]; thus, applying either PRP or PRF topically during and immediately after microneedling treatment can improve results by saturating the newly created fine, porous wounds with concentrated growth factors

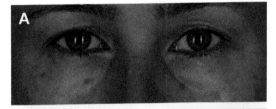

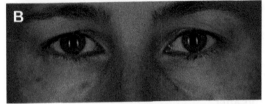

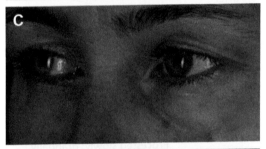

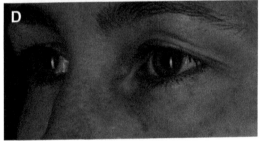

**Fig. 3.** (*A* and *C*) Before and (*B* and *D*) after 3 treatments of PRF alone injected to the infraorbital hollows of this 45-year-old female patient to correct pigmentation irregularities and provide subtle improvement in volumization.

(Video 2).[98] In 2 split-face studies comparing the effects of microneedling with topically applied vitamin C versus PRP, and distilled water versus PRP, respectively, the PRP-treated side showed better improvement in the presence of scars[103] and yielded improved overall skin texture,[104] more so than the respective non–PRP-treated side.

### Lasers

Laser resurfacing serves to retexturize the skin by stimulating the body's wound healing and tissue regeneration response. Topical application of PRP or PRF following such treatments may serve to both reduce healing time and enhance results by further supplementing the tissue injury

response with concentrated platele[t] multifunctional growth factors (**Fig.** face studies comparing the efficacy of [P]saline after fractional skin resurfacing, [?] treated side visually healed more rapidly t[han] saline-treated side.[105] Skin biopsies rev[ealed] improved collagen bundle thickness on the P[?]treated side compared with the saline-treate[d] side.[106] Although the complementary effects of PRF with ablative lasers have yet to undergo extensive analysis, anecdotal evidence in author K.K.'s practice suggests that PRF may yield similar, if not superior, benefits after laser resurfacing because of its prolonged growth factor release.

## FUTURE DIRECTIONS

Further research on PRP and PRF is warranted to better elucidate their functional roles in medical cosmetic rejuvenation. Although PRP has a more extensive history of applied use, research on the functionality and sustainability of growth factors and other regenerative cells in purely autologous PRF justifies its continued use. Comparative studies including both treatments may provide

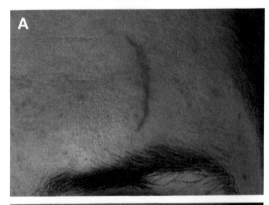

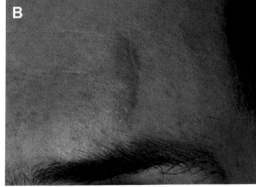

**Fig. 4.** (*A*) Before and (*B*) after 2 treatments of a fractionated laser combined with topical PRP to improve the presence of this 25-year-old male patient's forehead scar.

additional insight into the preferential implications of each.

### Platelet Therapies in Combination with Adipose-derived Stem Cells

PRF has been shown to enhance the proliferation of nanofat-derived stem cells in vitro in a dose-dependent manner.[107] ASCs cultured in PRP have also been shown to have stimulatory effects on the proliferation and migration of dermal fibroblasts and keratinocytes.[108] This finding suggests that ASCs support reepithelialization via paracrine pathways and help maintain epidermal homeostasis.[24]

These synergistic relationships found in vitro have been shown clinically. PRP has been shown to improve fat graft outcomes as a result of enhanced survival of fat cells and ASC differentiation triggered by the growth factors present in PRP.[109] One study showed that patients who received nanofat, PRF, and autologous fat transplant showed improvement in soft tissue depression and skin texture along with high patient satisfaction compared with traditional autologous fat transplant.[110] Another study compared nanofat and intradermal PRF injection with hyaluronic acid injection. Facial skin texture was improved to a greater extent and there was a higher satisfaction rate in the nanofat-PRF group.[107] Gentile and colleagues[30] found that both fat grafts enriched with SVF and fat grafts enriched with PRP were effective at improving facial scars and maintaining contour restoration and lower fat resorption after 1 year, compared with controls who received centrifuged fat injections without SVF or PRP.

### Other Autologous Cell Types

Other autologous therapies, such as fibroblasts, keratinocytes, dermal papillae, and melanocytes, have also been developed for various cosmetic and medical purposes.[111] Autologous fibroblasts, in particular, are used for aesthetic purposes. Dermal fibroblasts are mesenchymal cells that synthesize collagen and glycosaminoglycans and are involved in cutaneous wound healing and skin repair.[112]

Autologous cultured fibroblasts are injected into the patient's dermis with resulting long-lasting filling effect up to 48 months, thought to be caused by continuous protein repair.[113–115] Laviv (Fibrocell Technologies, Inc, Exton, PA) has been approved for use in nasolabial folds; however, 3 treatment sessions every 3 to 6 weeks are required and the fibroblasts are sourced through a postauricular biopsy.[116,117] However, 1 study that used Laviv in the nasojugal groove

showed improvement after 1 session compared with placebo without any serious adverse events.[118]

## OTHER NOVEL SKIN REJUVENATION THERAPIES

Although autologous therapies have great potential for skin rejuvenation, traditional minimally invasive cosmetic procedures continue to dominate the aesthetic industry.[1,119] New developments in botulinum toxin, fillers, threads, and combination therapies are discussed next.

### Neurotoxins

Botulinum toxin type A (BoNTA) injections using products such as Botox (onabotulinumtoxinA), Dysport (abobotulinumtoxinA), and Xeomin (incobotulinumtoxinA) continue to be the most popular noninvasive cosmetic procedures and their popularity continues to increase.[1,119]

New neurotoxin products and techniques are entering the sphere of facial rejuvenation. Jeuveau (prabotulinumtoxinA-xvfs) (Evolus, Inc, Irvine, CA), a low-cost alternative to other neurotoxins, has been approved by the FDA for treatment of glabellar lines.[120,121] DaxibotulinumtoxinA, a neurotoxin developed by Revance Therapeutics (Newark, CA), is a long-acting product formulated with a proprietary peptide that was found to be safe and effective for moderate or severe glabellar lines in phase 2 and 3 studies.[122,123]

Originally approved for correcting wrinkles of the glabella and the periorbital region, the extensive off-label use of BoNTA in different areas of the face is now expanding to different methods of delivery.[124,125] The microbotox method was developed to provide a more natural look for patients, with effects lasting up to 6 months.[126] Highly diluted onabotulinumtoxinA is injected in multiple small blebs at 0.8-cm to 1.0-cm intervals into the dermis or the interface between the dermis and the superficial surface of the muscles of the face and neck. This more superficial approach is thought to prevent a frozen appearance while also improving skin texture because of atrophy of sebaceous and sweat glands.

A recent study compared the intramuscular injection versus intradermal microdroplets injection versus nanomicroneedle delivery of BoNTA for the treatment of crow's feet.[127] For dynamic wrinkles, intramuscular injection and intradermal microdroplet injections were more effective than nanomicroneedles. For static wrinkles, nanomicroneedles and intradermal microdroplets injection were more effective. Skin elasticity, collagen content, and hydration of nanomicroneedle group and intradermal microdroplet group increased more significantly than those of the intramuscular injection group and were highest at 12 weeks in the intradermal microdroplet group.

There are some limited data supporting the use of BoNTA for hypertrophic scars and keloids, but further studies are required to evaluate BoNTA in wound healing and scarring.[128,129]

## Fillers

The growing popularity of injectable fillers follows behind the popularity of neurotoxins. Most fillers used on the market now are absorbable fillers made up of either hyaluronic acid, polylactic acid, hydroxylapatite calcium microspheres, or collagen. Ellansé (Sinclair Pharmaceuticals, London, United Kingdom), composed of polycaprolactone microspheres in an aqueous carboxymethylcellulose gel carrier, is a collagen biostimulator with results lasting up to 4 years in certain product lines.[130] Bellafill (Suneva Medical, Inc, Santa Barbara, CA), consists of 80% bovine collagen gel and 20% polymethylmethacrylate (PMMA) microspheres, forming a matrix that supports the production of endogenous collagen over time.[131] Silk Medical Aesthetics Inc has developed a biocompatible liquid silk filler made from pure silk from the thread of silkworm cocoons that will be undergoing clinical trials soon.[132]

Diluted calcium hydroxylapatite (CaHA) has also recently been used for skin tightening purposes in individuals who have age-associated upper arm skin changes.[133] CaHA's microspheres have been shown to stimulate fibroblast proliferation neocollagenesis, neoelastogenesis, and angiogenesis.[133–135] Diluted CaHA is also used in the neck and décolletage to stimulate neocollagenesis by a procedure using multiple retrograde linear threading passes of diluted CaHA in the subdermal plane followed by massage with a gel or cream.[133]

An advanced injection technique called myomodulation has also recently been introduced in the scientific literature.[136] The clinician addresses muscle movement with injectable fillers in the treatment of facial structural deficiencies by supporting muscle movement or blocking overaction. These effects can be augmented with neurotoxins, highlighting the importance of individualized, combination therapies when rejuvenating the skin.

## Thread Lifts

The placement of dissolvable sutures continues to gain popularity as a minimally invasive treatment of facial ptosis that provides a temporary lifting of drooping tissues with a low risk of complications.

Dissolvable barbed sutures, most commonly made of polydioxanone (PDO), are placed under the skin of the face and neck to reduce skin laxity, creating a brow, midface, jawline, and chin and/or neck lift, while also stimulating collagen formation[137–140] (**Fig. 5**). Suspension threads, which contain barbs, have the added benefit of stimulating collagen formation. On histology, fibrous capsules have been found along threads, which are thought to contribute to lifting surrounding tissues.[1–3] This fibrosis, associated with acute inflammatory cells, is eventually replaced by type I collagen.[4–6]

Skin rejuvenation and facial skin lifting results achieved with threads have been noted for up to 24 months.[138] However, combination therapy with dermal fillers can improve the long-term results by compounding the effects of neocollagenesis.[141] In order to further maximize results, it is also important to carefully select patients with adequate tissue volume and for the procedure to be performed by a skilled clinician.[137,142] Lifting of ptotic tissues with PDO threads is best recommended for patients with contraindications to invasive surgical procedures, those who are amenable to short-term results for a lower cost, or those who combine the procedure with other modalities such as dermal fillers.[138]

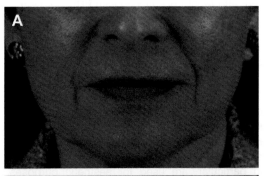
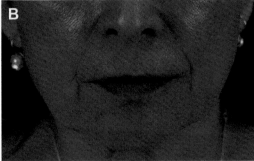

**Fig. 5.** (*A*) Before and (*B*) 4 months after midface PDO thread lift. Two threads were placed on each side. Improvement of nasiolabial folds is apparent.

Nevertheless, advancements continue to be made with this technology, with several thread types available, from free-standing, barbed threads that do not need to be suspended to smooth threads that need to be anchored to a stable structure of the face or scalp.

## Combination Treatments

Given that aging involves changes not only in the skin and fat but also bones, muscles, and ligaments, rejuvenation techniques must address each component of the aging process. A one-size-fits-all technique only using one modality is not as effective as a treatment plan that is tailored to the individual's needs using combination therapy, all while meeting the patient's goals and expectations. Although many of these therapies are not new, the concept of combining therapies is being emphasized in clinical practice (**Fig. 6**).

Combination therapies (**Table 4**) can potentially achieve better, quicker results at a lower cost to the patient with high patient satisfaction.[143–151] For example, accordion lines can be treated using superficial injections or microneedling application of highly diluted BoNTA and non–cross-linked hyaluronic acid.[143,152,153] It is important to also tailor therapies to the individual, such as taking an individual's ethnicity features into consideration. It is also crucial to remember that skin rejuvenation also applies to areas other than the face affected

| Table 4 | |
|---|---|
| **Combination therapies in aesthetic medicine** | |
| **Modality** | **Purpose** |
| Ablative lasers Collagen-stimulating treatments PRP/PRF Microneedling Radiofrequency/ ultrasound Microdermabrasion Skin peels Topical therapies; eg, retinol and hydroquinone | Reverse skin sagging and dullness Correct pigmentation |
| Botulinum toxin | Correct dynamic wrinkles |
| Fillers: Hyaluronic acid filler Calcium hydroxylapatite filler Poly-L-lactic acid filler Autologous fat tissue | Volume augmentation |

by aging, including the neck, décolletage, and the hands.

## SUMMARY

The rapidly growing aesthetic industry is continuously evolving to meet the increasing demand for cosmetic enhancement. With this expansion has come new technology within regenerative medicine, providing natural, effective, and safe skin rejuvenation. Using a combination approach, new innovations in injectable botulinum toxin and fillers, along with state-of-the-art autologous stem cells, lipofilling, and platelet therapies, can help patients reach their aesthetic goals.

## SUPPLEMENTARY DATA

Supplementary data related to this article can be found online at https://doi.org/10.1016/j.fsc.2019.09.009.

## REFERENCES

1. AAFPRS 2018 Annual survey reveals key trends in facial plastic surgery. 2019. Available at: https://www.aafprs.org/media/stats_polls/m_stats.html. Accessed March 20, 2019.
2. Nowacki M, Kloskowski T, Pietkun K, et al. The use of stem cells in aesthetic dermatology and plastic surgery procedures. A compact review of

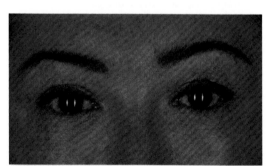
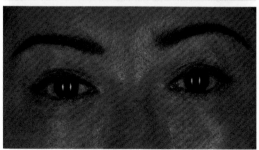

**Fig. 6.** (*Top*) Before and (*bottom*) after views of a patient who received injections of PRF mixed with dermal filler under both eyes.

experimental and clinical applications. Postepy Dermatol Alergol 2017;34(6):526–34.

3. Zhu X, Du J, Liu G. The comparison of multilineage differentiation of bone marrow and adipose-derived mesenchymal stem cells. Clin Lab 2012; 58(9–10):897–903.

4. Brzoska M, Geiger H, Gauer S, et al. Epithelial differentiation of human adipose tissue-derived adult stem cells. Biochem Biophys Res Commun 2005; 330(1):142–50.

5. Cao Y, Sun Z, Liao L, et al. Human adipose tissue-derived stem cells differentiate into endothelial cells in vitro and improve postnatal neovascularization in vivo. Biochem Biophys Res Commun 2005; 332(2):370–9.

6. Kapur SK, Dos-Anjos Vilaboa S, Llull R, et al. Adipose tissue and stem/progenitor cells: discovery and development. Clin Plast Surg 2015;42(2): 155–67.

7. Conde-Green A, Marano AA, Lee ES, et al. Fat grafting and adipose-derived regenerative cells in burn wound healing and scarring: a systematic review of the literature. Plast Reconstr Surg 2016; 137(1):302–12.

8. Zuk PA, Zhu M, Mizuno H, et al. Multilineage cells from human adipose tissue: implications for cell-based therapies. Tissue Eng 2001;7(2):211–28.

9. Rosenthal T. Calcium antagonists in the treatment of severe refractory hypertension. J Cardiovasc Pharmacol 1988;12(Suppl 6):S93–7.

10. Kluth SM, Radke TF, Kogler G. Potential application of cord blood-derived stromal cells in cellular therapy and regenerative medicine. J Blood Transfus 2012;2012:365182.

11. Kalaszczynska I, Ferdyn K. Wharton's jelly derived mesenchymal stem cells: future of regenerative medicine? Recent findings and clinical significance. Biomed Res Int 2015;2015:430847.

12. Harris DT. Umbilical cord tissue mesenchymal stem cells: characterization and clinical applications. Curr Stem Cell Res Ther 2013;8(5):394–9.

13. Gimble JM, Katz AJ, Bunnell BA. Adipose-derived stem cells for regenerative medicine. Circ Res 2007;100(9):1249–60.

14. Raposio E, Caruana G, Petrella M, et al. A standardized method of isolating adipose-derived stem cells for clinical applications. Ann Plast Surg 2016;76(1):124–6.

15. Raposio E, Caruana G, Bonomini S, et al. A novel and effective strategy for the isolation of adipose-derived stem cells: minimally manipulated adipose-derived stem cells for more rapid and safe stem cell therapy. Plast Reconstr Surg 2014; 133(6):1406–9.

16. Shridharani SM, Broyles JM, Matarasso A. Liposuction devices: technology update. Med Devices (Auckl) 2014;7:241–51.

17. Halvorsen YC, Wilkison WO, Gimble JM. Adipose-derived stromal cells–their utility and potential in bone formation. Int J Obes Relat Metab Disord 2000;24(Suppl 4):S41–4.

18. Rodbell M. Metabolism of isolated fat cells. I. Effects of hormones on glucose metabolism and lipolysis. J Biol Chem 1964;239:375–80.

19. Ong WK, Sugii S. Adipose-derived stem cells: fatty potentials for therapy. Int J Biochem Cell Biol 2013; 45(6):1083–6.

20. Tonnard P, Verpaele A, Peeters G, et al. Nanofat grafting: basic research and clinical applications. Plast Reconstr Surg 2013;132(4):1017–26.

21. Tang W, Zeve D, Suh JM, et al. White fat progenitor cells reside in the adipose vasculature. Science 2008;322(5901):583–6.

22. Blanpain C, Horsley V, Fuchs E. Epithelial stem cells: turning over new leaves. Cell 2007;128(3): 445–58.

23. Blanpain C, Fuchs E. Epidermal homeostasis: a balancing act of stem cells in the skin. Nat Rev Mol Cell Biol 2009;10(3):207–17.

24. Gaur M, Dobke M, Lunyak VV. Mesenchymal stem cells from adipose tissue in clinical applications for dermatological indications and skin aging. Int J Mol Sci 2017;18(1) [pii:E208].

25. Cappuzzello C, Doni A, Dander E, et al. Mesenchymal stromal cell-derived PTX3 promotes wound healing via fibrin remodeling. J Invest Dermatol 2016;136(1):293–300.

26. Festa E, Fretz J, Berry R, et al. Adipocyte lineage cells contribute to the skin stem cell niche to drive hair cycling. Cell 2011;146(5):761–71.

27. Dernbach E, Urbich C, Brandes RP, et al. Antioxidative stress-associated genes in circulating progenitor cells: evidence for enhanced resistance against oxidative stress. Blood 2004;104(12): 3591–7.

28. Cousin B, Munoz O, Andre M, et al. A role for pre-adipocytes as macrophage-like cells. FASEB J 1999;13(2):305–12.

29. Cousin B, Andre M, Casteilla L, et al. Altered macrophage-like functions of preadipocytes in inflammation and genetic obesity. J Cell Physiol 2001;186(3):380–6.

30. Gentile P, De Angelis B, Pasin M, et al. Adipose-derived stromal vascular fraction cells and platelet-rich plasma: basic and clinical evaluation for cell-based therapies in patients with scars on the face. J Craniofac Surg 2014; 25(1):267–72.

31. Wang M, Crisostomo PR, Herring C, et al. Human progenitor cells from bone marrow or adipose tissue produce VEGF, HGF, and IGF-I in response to TNF by a p38 MAPK-dependent mechanism. Am J Physiol Regul Integr Comp Physiol 2006; 291(4):R880–4.

32. Rehman J, Traktuev D, Li J, et al. Secretion of angiogenic and antiapoptotic factors by human adipose stromal cells. Circulation 2004;109(10):1292–8.

33. Garcia-Olmo D, Garcia-Arranz M, Herreros D, et al. A phase I clinical trial of the treatment of Crohn's fistula by adipose mesenchymal stem cell transplantation. Dis Colon Rectum 2005;48(7):1416–23.

34. Salgado AJ, Reis RL, Sousa NJ, et al. Adipose tissue derived stem cells secretome: soluble factors and their roles in regenerative medicine. Curr Stem Cell Res Ther 2010;5(2):103–10.

35. Yun IS, Jeon YR, Lee WJ, et al. Effect of human adipose derived stem cells on scar formation and remodeling in a pig model: a pilot study. Dermatol Surg 2012;38(10):1678–88.

36. Jeong JH, Fan Y, You GY, et al. Improvement of photoaged skin wrinkles with cultured human fibroblasts and adipose-derived stem cells: a comparative study. J Plast Reconstr Aesthet Surg 2015;68(3):372–81.

37. Zhang S, Dong Z, Peng Z, et al. Anti-aging effect of adipose-derived stem cells in a mouse model of skin aging induced by D-galactose. PLoS One 2014;9(5):e97573.

38. Sung HM, Suh IS, Lee HB, et al. Case reports of adipose-derived stem cell therapy for nasal skin necrosis after filler injection. Arch Plast Surg 2012;39(1):51–4.

39. Kim JH, Ahn DK, Jeong HS, et al. Treatment algorithm of complications after filler injection: based on wound healing process. J Korean Med Sci 2014;29(Suppl 3):S176–82.

40. Arshad Z, Halioua-Haubold CL, Roberts M, et al. Adipose-derived stem cells in aesthetic surgery: a mixed methods evaluation of the current clinical trial, intellectual property, and regulatory landscape. Aesthet Surg J 2018;38(2):199–210.

41. Arnhold S, Klein H, Semkova I, et al. Neurally selected embryonic stem cells induce tumor formation after long-term survival following engraftment into the subretinal space. Invest Ophthalmol Vis Sci 2004;45(12):4251–5.

42. Herberts CA, Kwa MS, Hermsen HP. Risk factors in the development of stem cell therapy. J Transl Med 2011;9:29.

43. Fortin JM, Azari H, Zheng T, et al. Transplantation of defined populations of differentiated human neural stem cell progeny. Sci Rep 2016;6:23579.

44. Torsvik A, Rosland GV, Svendsen A, et al. Spontaneous malignant transformation of human mesenchymal stem cells reflects cross-contamination: putting the research field on track - letter. Cancer Res 2010;70(15):6393–6.

45. Rubio D, Garcia-Castro J, Martin MC, et al. Spontaneous human adult stem cell transformation. Cancer Res 2005;65(8):3035–9.

46. Wu W, Niklason L, Steinbacher DM. The effect of age on human adipose-derived stem cells. Plast Reconstr Surg 2013;131(1):27–37.

47. Bourin P, Bunnell BA, Casteilla L, et al. Stromal cells from the adipose tissue-derived stromal vascular fraction and culture expanded adipose tissue-derived stromal/stem cells: a joint statement of the International Federation for Adipose Therapeutics and Science (IFATS) and the International Society for Cellular Therapy (ISCT). Cytotherapy 2013;15(6):641–8.

48. Singer R, Nahai F. Regulation of stem-cell treatments: a problem that is only getting worse. Aesthet Surg J 2019;39(4):460–2.

49. Roh MR, Kim TK, Chung KY. Treatment of infraorbital dark circles by autologous fat transplantation: a pilot study. Br J Dermatol 2009;160(5):1022–5.

50. Boureaux E, Chaput B, Bannani S, et al. Eyelid fat grafting: Indications, operative technique and complications; a systematic review. J Craniomaxillofac Surg 2016;44(4):374–80.

51. Kakagia D, Pallua N. Autologous fat grafting: in search of the optimal technique. Surg Innov 2014;21(3):327–36.

52. Coleman SR, Katzel EB. Fat grafting for facial filling and regeneration. Clin Plast Surg 2015;42(3):289–300, vii.

53. Marten TJ, Elyassnia D. Fat grafting in facial rejuvenation. Clin Plast Surg 2015;42(2):219–52.

54. Sinno S, Mehta K, Reavey PL, et al. Current trends in facial rejuvenation: an assessment of ASPS Members' use of fat grafting during face lifting. Plast Reconstr Surg 2015;136(1):20e–30e.

55. Klinger M, Marazzi M, Vigo D, et al. Fat injection for cases of severe burn outcomes: a new perspective of scar remodeling and reduction. Aesthetic Plast Surg 2008;32(3):465–9.

56. Klinger M, Caviggioli F, Klinger FM, et al. Autologous fat graft in scar treatment. J Craniofac Surg 2013;24(5):1610–5.

57. Bernardini FP, Gennai A, Izzo L, et al. Superficial enhanced fluid fat injection (SEFFI) to correct volume defects and skin aging of the face and periocular region. Aesthet Surg J 2015;35(5):504–15.

58. Gennai A, Zambelli A, Repaci E, et al. Skin rejuvenation and volume enhancement with the micro superficial enhanced fluid fat injection (M-SEFFI) for skin aging of the periocular and perioral regions. Aesthet Surg J 2017;37(1):14–23.

59. Khouri RK, Smit JM, Cardoso E, et al. Percutaneous aponeurotomy and lipofilling: a regenerative alternative to flap reconstruction? Plast Reconstr Surg 2013;132(5):1280–90.

60. Simonacci F, Bertozzi N, Grieco MP, et al. Procedure, applications, and outcomes of autologous fat grafting. Ann Med Surg (Lond) 2017;20:49–60.

61. Moscatello DK, Schiavi J, Marquart JD, et al. Collagenase-assisted fat dissociation for autologous fat transfer. Dermatol Surg 2008;34(10):1314–21 [discussion: 1321–2].

62. Piasecki JH, Gutowski KA, Lahvis GP, et al. An experimental model for improving fat graft viability and purity. Plast Reconstr Surg 2007;119(5):1571–83.

63. Youn S, Shin JI, Kim JD, et al. Correction of infraorbital dark circles using collagenase-digested fat cell grafts. Dermatol Surg 2013;39(5):766–72.

64. Nguyen PS, Desouches C, Gay AM, et al. Development of micro-injection as an innovative autologous fat graft technique: The use of adipose tissue as dermal filler. J Plast Reconstr Aesthet Surg 2012;65(12):1692–9.

65. Zeltzer AA, Tonnard PL, Verpaele AM. Sharp-needle intradermal fat grafting (SNIF). Aesthet Surg J 2012;32(5):554–61.

66. Jansma J, Schepers RH, Vissink A. Microfat transfer in cosmetic facial procedures. Ned Tijdschr Tandheelkd 2014;121(6):330–5 [in Dutch].

67. Mahdavian Delavary B, van der Veer WM, van Egmond M, et al. Macrophages in skin injury and repair. Immunobiology 2011;216(7):753–62.

68. Gu Z, Li Y, Li H. Use of condensed nanofat combined with fat grafts to treat atrophic scars. JAMA Facial Plast Surg 2018;20(2):128–35.

69. Yoshimura K, Sato K, Aoi N, et al. Cell-assisted lipotransfer for facial lipoatrophy: efficacy of clinical use of adipose-derived stem cells. Dermatol Surg 2008;34(9):1178–85.

70. Matsumoto D, Sato K, Gonda K, et al. Cell-assisted lipotransfer: supportive use of human adipose-derived cells for soft tissue augmentation with lipoinjection. Tissue Eng 2006;12(12):3375–82.

71. Dohan Ehrenfest DM, Andia I, Zumstein MA, et al. Classification of platelet concentrates (Platelet-Rich Plasma-PRP, Platelet-Rich Fibrin-PRF) for topical and infiltrative use in orthopedic and sports medicine: current consensus, clinical implications and perspectives. Muscles Ligaments Tendons J 2014;4(1):3–9.

72. Marx RE, Carlson ER, Eichstaedt RM, et al. Platelet-rich plasma: growth factor enhancement for bone grafts. Oral Surg Oral Med Oral Pathol Oral Radiol Endod 1998;85(6):638–46.

73. Choukroun J, Adda F, Schoeffer C, et al. PRF: an opportunity in perio-implantology. Implantodontie 2000;41:55–62.

74. Barrientos S, Stojadinovic O, Golinko MS, et al. Growth factors and cytokines in wound healing. Wound Repair Regen 2008;16(5):585–601.

75. Fabi S, Sundaram H. The potential of topical and injectable growth factors and cytokines for skin rejuvenation. Facial Plast Surg 2014;30(2):157–71.

76. Sundaram H, Mehta RC, Norine JA, et al. Topically applied physiologically balanced growth factors: a new paradigm of skin rejuvenation. J Drugs Dermatol 2009;8(5 Suppl Skin Rejuenation):4–13.

77. Garg AK. Autologous blood concentrates. Batavia (IL): Quintessence Publishing Co. Inc; 2018.

78. de Boer HC, Verseyden C, Ulfman LH, et al. Fibrin and activated platelets cooperatively guide stem cells to a vascular injury and promote differentiation towards an endothelial cell phenotype. Arterioscler Thromb Vasc Biol 2006;26(7):1653–9.

79. Ponte AL, Marais E, Gallay N, et al. The in vitro migration capacity of human bone marrow mesenchymal stem cells: comparison of chemokine and growth factor chemotactic activities. Stem Cells 2007;25(7):1737–45.

80. Mescher AL. Junqueira's basic histology text & atlas. 15 edition. New York: McGraw-Hill; 2013.

81. Brummel KE, Butenas S, Mann KG. An integrated study of fibrinogen during blood coagulation. J Biol Chem 1999;274(32):22862–70.

82. Mann KG, Brummel K, Butenas S. What is all that thrombin for? J Thromb Haemost 2003;1(7):1504–14.

83. Undas A, Ariens RA. Fibrin clot structure and function: a role in the pathophysiology of arterial and venous thromboembolic diseases. Arterioscler Thromb Vasc Biol 2011;31(12):e88–99.

84. Fujioka-Kobayashi M, Miron RJ, Hernandez M, et al. Optimized platelet-rich fibrin with the low-speed concept: growth factor release, biocompatibility, and cellular response. J Periodontol 2017;88(1):112–21.

85. Kobayashi E, Fluckiger L, Fujioka-Kobayashi M, et al. Comparative release of growth factors from PRP, PRF, and advanced-PRF. Clin Oral Investig 2016;20(9):2353–60.

86. Dohan Ehrenfest DM, Rasmusson L, Albrektsson T. Classification of platelet concentrates: from pure platelet-rich plasma (P-PRP) to leucocyte- and platelet-rich fibrin (L-PRF). Trends Biotechnol 2009;27(3):158–67.

87. Giannini S, Cielo A, Bonanome L, et al. Comparison between PRP, PRGF and PRF: lights and shadows in three similar but different protocols. Eur Rev Med Pharmacol Sci 2015;19(6):927–30.

88. Utomo DN, Mahyudin F, Hernugrahanto KD, et al. Implantation of platelet rich fibrin and allogenic mesenchymal stem cells facilitate the healing of muscle injury: an experimental study on animal. International Journal of Surgery Open 2018;11:4–9.

89. Zenker S. Platelet rich plasma (PRP) for facial rejuvenation. J Méd Esthet Chir Derm 2010;XXXVII(148):179–83.

90. Dohan Ehrenfest DM, de Peppo GM, Doglioli P, et al. Slow release of growth factors and thrombospondin-1 in Choukroun's platelet-rich

fibrin (PRF): a gold standard to achieve for all surgical platelet concentrates technologies. Growth Factors 2009;27(1):63–9.

91. Ghanaati S, Booms P, Orlowska A, et al. Advanced platelet-rich fibrin: a new concept for cell-based tissue engineering by means of inflammatory cells. J Oral Implantol 2014;40(6):679–89.

92. Masuki H, Okudera T, Watanebe T, et al. Growth factor and pro-inflammatory cytokine contents in platelet-rich plasma (PRP), plasma rich in growth factors (PRGF), advanced platelet-rich fibrin (A-PRF), and concentrated growth factors (CGF). Int J Implant Dent 2016;2(1):19.

93. Di Liddo R, Bertalot T, Borean A, et al. Leucocyte and platelet-rich fibrin: a carrier of autologous multipotent cells for regenerative medicine. J Cell Mol Med 2018;22(3):1840–54.

94. Abd El Raouf M, Wang X, Miusi S, et al. Injectable-platelet rich fibrin using the low speed centrifugation concept improves cartilage regeneration when compared to platelet-rich plasma. Platelets 2019;30(2):213–21.

95. Naik B, Karunakar P, Jayadev M, et al. Role of Platelet rich fibrin in wound healing: a critical review. J Conserv Dent 2013;16(4):284–93.

96. He L, Lin Y, Hu X, et al. A comparative study of platelet-rich fibrin (PRF) and platelet-rich plasma (PRP) on the effect of proliferation and differentiation of rat osteoblasts in vitro. Oral Surg Oral Med Oral Pathol Oral Radiol Endod 2009;108(5): 707–13.

97. Karimi K, Rockwell H. The benefits of platelet rich fibrin (PRF). Facial Plast Surg Clin North Am 2019;27(3):331–40.

98. Puri N. Platelet rich plasma in dermatology and aesthetic medicine. Our Dermatology Online 2015;6(2):207–11.

99. Farage MA, Miller KW, Elsner P, et al. Characteristics of the aging skin. Adv Wound Care (New Rochelle) 2013;2(1):5–10.

100. Kim DH, Je YJ, Kim CD, et al. Can Platelet-rich plasma be used for skin rejuvenation? Evaluation of effects of platelet-rich plasma on human dermal fibroblast. Ann Dermatol 2011;23(4):424–31.

101. Aust MC, Fernandes D, Kolokythas P, et al. Percutaneous collagen induction therapy: an alternative treatment for scars, wrinkles, and skin laxity. Plast Reconstr Surg 2008;121(4):1421–9.

102. Fitzpatrick RE, Rostan EF. Reversal of photodamage with topical growth factors: a pilot study. J Cosmet Laser Ther 2003;5(1):25–34.

103. Chawla S. Split face comparative study of microneedling with PRP versus microneedling with vitamin C in treating atrophic post acne scars. J Cutan Aesthet Surg 2014;7(4):209–12.

104. Asif M, Kanodia S, Singh K. Combined autologous platelet-rich plasma with microneedling verses microneedling with distilled water in the treatment of atrophic acne scars: a concurrent split-face study. J Cosmet Dermatol 2016;15(4):434–43.

105. Lee JW, Kim BJ, Kim MN, et al. The efficacy of autologous platelet rich plasma combined with ablative carbon dioxide fractional resurfacing for acne scars: a simultaneous split-face trial. Dermatol Surg 2011;37(7):931–8.

106. Na JI, Choi JW, Choi HR, et al. Rapid healing and reduced erythema after ablative fractional carbon dioxide laser resurfacing combined with the application of autologous platelet-rich plasma. Dermatol Surg 2011;37(4):463–8.

107. Liang ZJ, Lu X, Li DQ, et al. Precise intradermal injection of nanofat-derived stromal cells combined with platelet-rich fibrin improves the efficacy of facial skin rejuvenation. Cell Physiol Biochem 2018;47(1):316–29.

108. Stessuk T, Puzzi MB, Chaim EA, et al. Platelet-rich plasma (PRP) and adipose-derived mesenchymal stem cells: stimulatory effects on proliferation and migration of fibroblasts and keratinocytes in vitro. Arch Dermatol Res 2016;308(7):511–20.

109. Modarressi A. Platlet rich plasma (PRP) improves fat grafting outcomes. World J Plast Surg 2013; 2(1):6–13.

110. Wei H, Gu SX, Liang YD, et al. Nanofat-derived stem cells with platelet-rich fibrin improve facial contour remodeling and skin rejuvenation after autologous structural fat transplantation. Oncotarget 2017;8(40):68542–56.

111. Kumar S, Mahajan BB, Kaur S, et al. Autologous therapies in dermatology. J Clin Aesthet Dermatol 2014;7(12):38–45.

112. Thangapazham RL, Darling TN, Meyerle J. Alteration of skin properties with autologous dermal fibroblasts. Int J Mol Sci 2014;15(5):8407–27.

113. Weiss RA, Weiss MA, Beasley KL, et al. Autologous cultured fibroblast injection for facial contour deformities: a prospective, placebo-controlled, Phase III clinical trial. Dermatol Surg 2007;33(3): 263–8.

114. Watson D, Keller GS, Lacombe V, et al. Autologous fibroblasts for treatment of facial rhytids and dermal depressions. A pilot study. Arch Facial Plast Surg 1999;1(3):165–70.

115. Boss WK Jr, Usal H, Chernoff G, et al. Autologous cultured fibroblasts as cellular therapy in plastic surgery. Clin Plast Surg 2000;27(4):613–26.

116. Schmidt C. FDA approves first cell therapy for wrinkle-free visage. Nat Biotechnol 2011;29(8): 674–5.

117. Smith SR, Munavalli G, Weiss R, et al. A multicenter, double-blind, placebo-controlled trial of autologous fibroblast therapy for the treatment of nasolabial fold wrinkles. Dermatol Surg 2012;38(7 Pt 2):1234–43.

118. Moon KC, Lee HS, Han SK, et al. Correcting naso-jugal groove with autologous cultured fibroblast injection: a pilot study. Aesthetic Plast Surg 2018; 42(3):815–24.

119. 2018 National Plastic Surgery Statistics. 2019. Available at: https://www.plasticsurgery.org/documents/News/Statistics/2018/plastic-surgery-statistics-report-2018.pdf. Accessed March 15, 2019.

120. Center for Drug Evaluation and Research Application Number: 761085Orig1s000. Available at: https://www.accessdata.fda.gov/drugsatfda_docs/nda/2019/761085Orig1s000OtherR.pdf. Accessed March 20, 2019.

121. JEUVEAU- prabotulinum toxin type a powder. Available at: https://dailymed.nlm.nih.gov/dailymed/drugInfo.cfm?setid=17a914c1-e54b-4b50-965d-b0fd9111bba4. Accessed March 20, 2019.

122. Two phase 3, randomized, double-blind, placebo-controlled, multicenter trials to evaluate the efficacy and safety of daxibotulinumtoxinA for injection to treat moderate to severe glabellar lines (SAKURA 1 and 2). J Am Acad Dermatol 2018;79(3):AB306.

123. Carruthers J, Solish N, Humphrey S, et al. Injectable daxibotulinumtoxina for the treatment of glabellar lines: a phase 2, randomized, dose-ranging, double-blind, multicenter comparison with onabotulinumtoxina and placebo. Dermatol Surg 2017;43(11):1321–31.

124. Carruthers J, Fournier N, Kerscher M, et al. The convergence of medicine and neurotoxins: a focus on botulinum toxin type A and its application in aesthetic medicine–a global, evidence-based botulinum toxin consensus education initiative: part II: incorporating botulinum toxin into aesthetic clinical practice. Dermatol Surg 2013;39(3 Pt 2): 510–25.

125. Erickson BP, Lee WW, Cohen J, et al. The role of neurotoxins in the periorbital and midfacial areas. Facial Plast Surg Clin North Am 2015;23(2):243–55.

126. Wu WT. Microbotox of the lower face and neck: evolution of a personal technique and its clinical effects. Plast Reconstr Surg 2015;136(5 Suppl): 92S–100S.

127. Cao Y, Yang JP, Zhu XG, et al. A comparative in vivo study on three treatment approaches to applying topical botulinum toxin A for crow's feet. Biomed Res Int 2018;2018:6235742.

128. Fanous A, Bezdjian A, Caglar D, et al. Treatment of keloid scars with botulinum toxin type A versus triamcinolone in an athymic nude mouse model. Plast Reconstr Surg 2019;143(3):760–7.

129. Campanati A, Martina E, Giuliodori K, et al. Botulinum toxin off-label use in dermatology: a review. Skin Appendage Disord 2017;3(1):39–56.

130. de Melo F, Nicolau P, Piovano L, et al. Recommendations for volume augmentation and rejuvenation of the face and hands with the new generation polycaprolactone-based collagen stimulator (Ellansé®). Clin Cosmet Investig Dermatol 2017;10:431–40.

131. Gold MH, Sadick NS. Optimizing outcomes with polymethylmethacrylate fillers. J Cosmet Dermatol 2018;17(3):298–304.

132. Thomas E. Silk Inc. Develops sustainable injectable dermal filler. 2018. Available at: https://wwd.com/beauty-industry-news/products/silk-inc-sustainable-injectable-dermal-filler-1202939693/. Accessed March 26, 2019.

133. Fabi S, Pavicic T, Braz A, et al. Combined aesthetic interventions for prevention of facial ageing, and restoration and beautification of face and body. Clin Cosmet Investig Dermatol 2017;10:423–9.

134. Yutskovskaya Y, Kogan E, Leshunov E. A randomized, split-face, histomorphologic study comparing a volumetric calcium hydroxylapatite and a hyaluronic acid-based dermal filler. J Drugs Dermatol 2014;13(9):1047–52.

135. Yutskovskaya YA, Kogan EA. Improved neocollagenesis and skin mechanical properties after injection of diluted calcium hydroxylapatite in the neck and decolletage: a pilot study. J Drugs Dermatol 2017;16(1):68–74.

136. de Maio M. Myomodulation with Injectable fillers: an innovative approach to addressing facial muscle movement. Aesthetic Plast Surg 2018;42(3): 798–814.

137. Wu WT. Barbed sutures in facial rejuvenation. Aesthet Surg J 2004;24(6):582–7.

138. Ali YH. Two years' outcome of thread lifting with absorbable barbed PDO threads: Innovative score for objective and subjective assessment. J Cosmet Laser Ther 2018;20(1):41–9.

139. Rezaee Khiabanloo S, Jebreili R, Aalipour E, et al. Outcomes in thread lift for face and neck: a study performed with Silhouette Soft and Promo Happy Lift double needle, innovative and classic techniques. J Cosmet Dermatol 2019;18(1):84–93.

140. Yoon JH, Kim SS, Oh SM, et al. Tissue changes over time after polydioxanone thread insertion: an animal study with pigs. J Cosmet Dermatol 2019; 18(3):885–91.

141. Karimi K, Reivitis A. Lifting the lower face with an absorbable polydioxanone (PDO) thread. J Drugs Dermatol 2017;16(9):932–4.

142. Sulamanidze MA, Fournier PF, Paikidze TG, et al. Removal of facial soft tissue ptosis with special threads. Dermatol Surg 2002;28(5):367–71.

143. Schlessinger J, Gilbert E, Cohen JL, et al. New uses of abobotulinumtoxina in aesthetics. Aesthet Surg J 2017;37(suppl_1):S45–58.

144. Schlessinger J, Kenkel J, Werschler P. Further enhancement of facial appearance with a hydroquinone skin care system plus tretinoin in patients

previously treated with botulinum toxin type A. Aesthet Surg J 2011;31(5):529–39.

145. Ascher B, Fanchon C, Kanoun-Copy L, et al. A skincare containing retinol adenosine and hyaluronic acid optimises the benefits from a type A botulinum toxin injection. J Cosmet Laser Ther 2012;14(5):234–8.

146. Pavicic T, Few JW, Huber-Vorlander J. A novel, multi-step, combination facial rejuvenation procedure for treatment of the whole face with incobotulinumtoxinA, and two dermal fillers- calcium hydroxylapatite and a monophasic, polydensified hyaluronic acid filler. J Drugs Dermatol 2013;12(9):978–84.

147. Beer KR, Julius H, Dunn M, et al. Remodeling of periorbital, temporal, glabellar, and crow's feet areas with hyaluronic acid and botulinum toxin. J Cosmet Dermatol 2014;13(2):143–50.

148. Lorenc ZP, Daro-Kaftan E. Optimizing facial rejuvenation outcomes by combining poly-L-lactic acid, hyaluronic acid, calcium hydroxylapatite, and neurotoxins: two case studies. J Drugs Dermatol 2014; 13(2):191–5.

149. Rubin MG, Cox SE, Kaminer MS, et al. Correcting age-related changes in the face by use of injectable fillers and neurotoxins. Semin Cutan Med Surg 2014;33(4 Suppl):S81–4.

150. Molina B, David M, Jain R, et al. Patient satisfaction and efficacy of full-facial rejuvenation using a combination of botulinum toxin type A and hyaluronic acid filler. Dermatol Surg 2015;41(Suppl 1): S325–32.

151. Sundaram H, Liew S, Signorini M, et al. Global aesthetics consensus: hyaluronic acid fillers and botulinum toxin type A-recommendations for combined treatment and optimizing outcomes in diverse patient populations. Plast Reconstr Surg 2016; 137(5):1410–23.

152. Mole B. Scratched faces: treatment of dynamic facial wrinkles through the simultaneous combined use of botulinium toxin A and hyaluronic acid. Ann Chir Plast Esthet 2012;57(3):194–201 [in French].

153. Mole B. Accordion wrinkle treatment through the targeted use of botulinum toxin injections. Aesthetic Plast Surg 2014;38(2):419–28.

# Pre- and Postoperative Care for Interventional Skin Rejuvenation

Kaete A. Archer, MD[a], Paul J. Carniol, MD[b],*

## KEYWORDS

- Preoperative • Postoperative care • Skin rejuvenation

## KEY POINTS

- Laser resurfacing restores some of the histologic changes associated with photoaging.
- Fractional resurfacing gives many of the benefits of resurfacing with a shorter recovery period and lower incidence of complications.
- Extent and duration of erythema post resurfacing varies with the extent and type of resurfacing.
- There is controversy surrounding the use of prophylactic antibiotics.
- For deep resurfacing antiviral prophylaxis for herpes simplex virus is recommended.

## INTRODUCTION

Facial aging is a combination of descent of facial tissues, atrophy of fat compartments, bony remodeling, and photoaging/chronologic changes of the skin. Photoaging of the skin is clinically and histologically distinct from the genetically programmed aging process. Photoaging is due to UV-A and UV-B–generated free radicals that cause DNA mutations, structural and enzymatic protein alterations, and lipid peroxidation.[1] The chronologic aging process is characterized by atrophy of the skin.[2] Photoaged skin, however, is thicker than normal with wrinkling, roughness, sallowness, telangiectasia, mottled hyperpigmentation, and a loss of elasticity.[3] Histologically, these changes represent a thickened, basket-woven stratum corneum, a thinner atrophic epidermis with atypia, irregular dispersion of melanin, decreased glycosaminoglycans, and abnormal elastic fibers in the dermis (solar elastosis).[4]

## ROLE OF RHYTIDECTOMY

A rhytidectomy will address facial aging changes owing to laxity and gravity but will do little to improve fine rhytids and photoaging. In fact, if the skin is pulled too tightly during a face-lift to improve cutaneous rhytids, the face will appear overly tight and unnatural, and the patient is at higher risk for widened scars. Tension on the skin is subject to biologic creep and relaxation, so the rhytids in this situation will ultimately reappear. This situation is particularly the case as the collagen and elastic fibers are not restored by these procedures.

## LASER RESURFACING

To address collagen loss and photoaging, surgeons are incorporating resurfacing techniques, such as laser and chemical peels, for a more comprehensive approach to facial rejuvenation. Ablative laser resurfacing was introduced in the mid-1990s with the carbon dioxide ($CO_2$) laser.[5] The $CO_2$ laser wavelength is strongly absorbed by water, which is the most abundant chromophore in the skin and comprises approximately 70% of its total volume.[6] This laser was ideal for generalized superficial ablation, but if the tissue-dwell time exceeded the 1 millisecond thermal

Disclosures: None.
[a] Aesthetic Institute of Manhattan for Facial and Plastic Surgery, 460 Park Avenue, 17th Floor, New York, NY 10022, USA; [b] Rutgers New Jersey Medical School, 33 Overlook Road, Suite 401, Summit, NJ 070901, USA
* Corresponding author.
E-mail address: pcarniol@gmail.com

relaxation time of the cutaneous tissue, there could be increased complications.[6] Other important factors are the fluence, depth of resurfacing, and postlaser skin care. Related to the technique, thermal diffusion-related tissue injury could occur, causing pigment changes, fibrosis, and scarring. Meticulous technique was required to avoid these complications.[5]

## FRACTIONAL LASERS

To address these concerns, the next generation of lasers used a fractional mode. The first fractional lasers were nonablative because they did not vaporize the skin surface. These lasers were followed by fractional resurfacing lasers, which ablated portions of the skin surface. Fractional resurfacing was achieved through a pattern of thermal injury zones produced by the laser beams at specific depths in the dermis. The new $CO_2$ fractional lasers could deliver high peak fluences in less than 1 millisecond, which resulted in precisely removing thin layers of skin while leaving an acceptably narrow zone of residual thermal damage.[6] Because of healing

from adjacent nonlasered skin and diminished bulk dermal temperature elevation with fractional lasers, there was quicker recovery and healing. There was also a diminished risk of scarring and pigmentation changes. Fractionated laser resurfacing has been shown to significantly improve facial skin texture, lentigines, pore size, and rhytids (**Fig. 1**).

Initially, the practice of combining face-lifting with skin resurfacing was controversial. In 2002, Koch and Perkins[7] presented a case series of safely performing face-lift and simultaneous full-face $CO_2$ laser resurfacing. In 2012, Truswell[8] presented a case series of 42 patients who had full-face ablative fractional resurfacing with simultaneous face-lifting. There were no patients with hypopigmentation, infection, or skin necrosis. These articles emphasized that technique adjustments are important when combining lifting and resurfacing. These techniques include ensuring adequate flap thickness, decreasing laser energy, laser "feathering" over elevated tissues, and appropriate patient selection (**Figs. 2** and **3**).

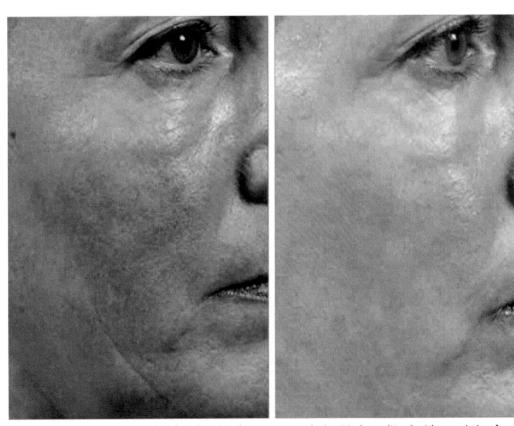

**Fig. 1.** Patient who underwent full-face fractional treatment with the $CO_2$ laser. (Used with permission from Carniol PJ, Hamilton M, Carniol ET. Current status of fractional laser resurfacing. *From JAMA Facial Plast Surg.* 2015;17(5):36-366; with permission.)

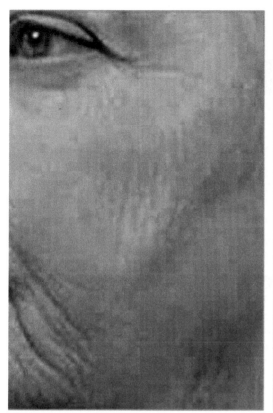 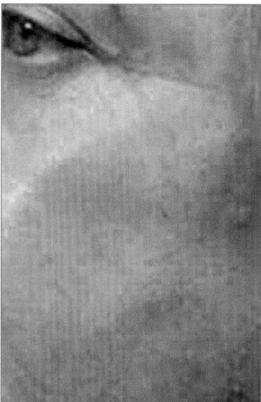

**Fig. 2.** Cheek skin following face-lift and full-face fractional $CO_2$ laser resurfacing. (Used with permission from Carniol PJ, Hamilton M, Carniol ET. Current status of fractional laser resurfacing. *From* JAMA Facial Plast Surg. 2015;17(5):36-366; with permission.)

## HISTOLOGIC EFFECTS OF LASER TREATMENTS

Resurfacing the skin with an ablative fractionated laser, such as the $CO_2$ or Erbium (Er), is an effective treatment of photoaging of the skin. At the histologic level, laser resurfacing results in the obliteration of the epidermis, partial ablation, or coagulative necrosis of the upper dermis along with wounding of the deeper skin regions.[9] Atypical, disorganized epidermal cells are replaced with normal well-organized cells.[9] Irregular, amorphous elastotic material in the superficial papillary dermis is replaced with normal compact collagen and elastin in regular, parallel alignment.[9]

## POSTRESURFACING ERYTHEMA

Erythema is expected after laser resurfacing. It can vary widely depending on the technology and technique. Frequently after fractional resurfacing, erythema is mild and well tolerated. Often it resolves within a few days. After nonfractional resurfacing, erythema lasts longer. The $CO_2$ laser can create greater thermal injury in the dermis compared with many Er-YAG lasers. Adjusting the pulse duration of an Er-YAG laser is used in some lasers to increase the benefits. Adjusting pulse duration results in a histologic result and inflammatory response similar to $CO_2$ laser. The risk for prolonged erythema is increased with the following factors: higher number of laser passes, tretinoin or glycolic acid use, and underlying rosacea.[10] Thermal stacking should also be avoided as, in addition to prolonged erythema, there is an associated risk of healing problems and scarring.

## LASER RESURFACING COMPLICATIONS

Optimization of postresurfacing management is important to diminish the risk of complications.

### Acne Outbreak/Dermatitis

Acne outbreaks may occur anywhere from 1 to 6 weeks after laser resurfacing. Acne can relate to postresurfacing skin care or the patient being prone to acne. Acne can particularly develop with postlaser prolonged occlusive skin care.

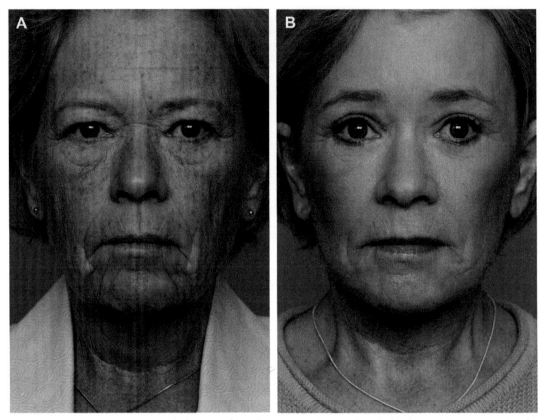

**Fig. 3.** (*A*) Preoperative patient with descent of facial tissues, jowling, and neck skin laxity. (*B*) Postoperative rhytidectomy with full-face $CO_2$ laser resurfacing. Patient shown is patient of senior author (S.W.P.). (*From* Archer KA, Perkins SW. Skin Resurfacing in Combination with Facelift Surgery. *Facial Plast Surg* 2017;33(3):299–310; with permission.)

### Infection

The most common viral infection after laser resurfacing is herpes simplex virus.[11] Despite prophylaxis, 2% to 7% of patients experience a herpetic outbreak.[10] Even patients with no history of herpetic outbreak can experience an active infection before reepithelialization is complete.[9] The most common bacterial infections are streptococcus, staphylococcus, and pseudomonas.[10]

### Postinflammatory Hyperpigmentation and Hypopigmentation

The most common adverse effect after laser resurfacing is postinflammatory hyperpigmentation, which can be seen in up to 33% of patients[10] (**Fig. 4**). A mild degree may be seen in the first month but will resolve by 3 months. Hypopigmentation can be seen 6 to 12 months following laser resurfacing. Hypopigmentation may relate to diminished dermal melanocytes.

### MINIMIZING COMPLICATIONS

Although it is not possible to avoid all complications, postlaser care can help to diminish the incidence of complications. There is still some controversy as to whether skin should be prepared for resurfacing. Initially skin preparation was thought to facilitate postresurfacing healing. More recently, many laser surgeons have stopped using a skin preparation regimen.

The exact skin-care protocols are dependent on the method of resurfacing and the depth of treatment. Differences in technology, laser technique, and ablation depths significantly affect the course of postoperative healing. Ablative, deeper treatments create more significant results than superficial treatments but have higher risk of complications and require more attention to preoperative and postoperative care.

### Prelaser Treatment Skin Care

Although a lack of consensus exists for certain aspects of the pretreatment regimen, the main goal

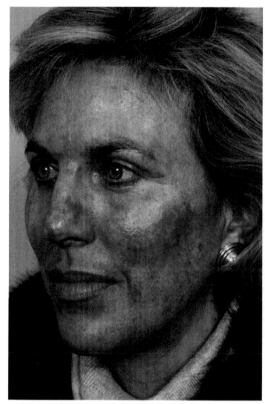

**Fig. 4.** Postinflammatory hyperpigmentation. (*From* Archer KA, Perkins SW. Skin Resurfacing in Combination with Facelift Surgery. *Facial Plast Surg* 2017;33(3):299–310; with permission.)

| Table 1 Fitzpatrick classification | | |
| --- | --- | --- |
| Skin Type | Skin Color | Tanning Characteristics |
| I | White | Always burns, never tans |
| II | White | Usually burns, tans less than average |
| III | White | Sometimes burns, average tan |
| IV | White | Rarely burns, tans more than average |
| V | Brown | Rarely burns, tans profusely |
| VI | Black | Never burns, marked pigment |

*Data from* Clark CP. Office-based skin care and superficial peels: the scientific rationale. Plast Reconstr Surg. 1999;104(3):854-864.

of pretreatment skin care is to increase the rate of epithelialization and decrease the risk of postinflammatory hyperpigmentation. Patients with higher Fitzpatrick skin types, because of increased melanin concentration, can have a higher incidence of postoperative dyschromia[12] (**Table 1**).[4]

Some laser surgeons favor using 4% hydroquinone daily to suppress the production of melanin, especially in patients with higher Fitzpatrick skin types. Hydroquinone inhibits tyrosinase, which inhibits the conversion of dopa to melanin.[13] It is hypothesized that decreasing the melanin content in the skin before resurfacing can decrease the rate of postinflammatory hyperpigmentation. Related to some controversy over the use of hydroquinone, other laser surgeons do not use it. Rather, they place their patients on strict sun precautions and avoid treating patients who are tanned. A controlled study of 100 patients with pretreatment topical tretinoin, hydroquinone, and/or glycolic acid indicated that pretreatment hydroquinone did not have a significant effect on posttreatment hyperpigmentation.[14] This lack of effect is likely because the epidermis is repopulated by

melanocytes originating from deep within the follicular unit.[14]

Many studies report that use of tretinoin cream before a resurfacing procedure can accelerate reepithelialization.[15–20] Beasley and colleagues[21] treated the skin on the backs of pigs with the Ultra-Pulse laser (Coherent Medical Group, Lumenis, Palo Alto, CA, USA). Half of each treatment site had been pretreated for 29 days with tretinoin cream 0.05%, and the other half received no pretreatment. The tretinoin-treated halves healed significantly faster than the nontreated control halves. In addition, the granular cell layer was thicker in the tretinoin group than the control group.

There are several factors to explain tretinoin's effect on wound healing. Retinoids increase mucopolysaccharides,[22] collagen,[23] and fibronectin synthesis.[24] Retinoids decrease collagenase production[25] and stimulate fibroblasts by increasing the number of available receptor sites for epidermal growth factor.[26]

In addition to tretinoin, patients can be scheduled for a glycolic acid peel 2 to 4 weeks before the laser treatment. Glycolic acid creams have been shown to reduce corneocyte cohesion, thin the stratum corneum, increase the rest of the epidermal thickness, and increase glycosaminoglycan and collagen production.[27,28]

## Early Postoperative Care

For nonablative fractional resurfacing, the skin care is minimal. A mild, hypoallergenic, fragrance-free cleanser and moisturizer for the first week after the laser procedure are recommended. Sun exposure should be avoided. When initial healing is completed, patients may resume their regular skin-care routine.

For patients undergoing ablative fractional resurfacing, the skin care is more involved, and stricter adherence is important. The laser-induced wound must be kept moist and clean, whether an open or closed technique of wound dressing is chosen. Partial-thickness cutaneous wounds heal faster and with a reduced risk of scarring if they are maintained in a moist environment. The presence of a dry crust or scab impedes keratinocyte migration.[9]

For fractional laser resurfacing, Aquaphor can be used to cover the entire laser treatment area (Beiersdorf Inc, Norwalk, CT, USA). As this can occlude skin pores, it is important to thoroughly remove the Aquaphor 2 to 4 times per day. After removal, the dilute acetic acid soaks are then applied on gauze for 15 to 30 minutes. The soaks can be made by adding 5 mL (1 teaspoonful) of white vinegar to 2 cups of water. Care should be taken to avoid back contaminating either the soak solution or the Aquaphor. In order to further reduce the risk of back contamination, the senior author advises patients to only use Aquaphor in a tube not in a tub. In addition to minimizing crust formation, the dilute acetic acid will help to debride the crusting and provide an antibacterial function.[12] The wound care regimen is continued until reepithelialization has been achieved. Depending on the resurfacing procedure, this can vary from 1 to 10 days postoperatively.

### Postepithelialization Skin Care

Once initial healing is completed, skin-care regimens vary. The senior author favors a simple regimen consisting of a hypoallergenic mild moisturizer, mineral-based makeup, sunscreen, and avoiding sun exposure. Some investigators favor application of a nonhalogenated corticosteroid after complete epithelialization has occurred, such as mometasone.[11] For areas of delayed healing, an occlusive hydrocolloid dressing may be placed and changed every 2 to 3 days until epithelialization is complete. Alternatively, the Aquaphor skin-care regimen can be used only to that area. It is imperative that the patient avoids direct sun exposure and uses sunscreen with a sun protection factor 30 or higher, as well as UV-A protection every day to avoid dyschromia. As long as there is even mild erythema, the patient needs to avoid direct sun exposure.

Prolonged erythema can be treated with a vascular laser to diminish the pinkness and/or a strong class I topical corticosteroid.[10] The routine use of postoperative oral corticosteroids to reduce facial edema may cause delayed wound healing, and the use should be carefully evaluated. Post-treatment use of topical tretinoin, glycolic acid, and hydroquinone, and periodic light glycolic acid peels can help reduce the duration and severity of postlaser hyperpigmentation. Hypopigmentation that remains can be difficult to treat. Topical glycolic acid 30% to 40% peel with a light 15% tricholoracetic acid peel can be used to blend the area.[10] Makeup will also help to cover and blend this type of dyspigmentation in the first few months of healing.

Acne outbreaks may be treated with tetracycline, erythromycin, or minocycline. Treatment of irritant dermatitis includes stopping the irritant and limiting topical dressings to Aquaphor or plain petroleum. Cold compresses, antihistamine, oral steroids, and a mild topical corticosteroid may be helpful as well.

## PROPHYLACTIC MEDICATION

Some aspects of prophylactic medication use are agreed upon, and others are more controversial. It is standard of care and essential to prescribe antiviral prophylaxis for deep resurfacing. As mentioned, approximately 2% to 7% of all laser resurfacing patients experience active infection with the herpes simplex virus, especially in the perioral area.[10,29–31] In their own series, Perkins and Sklarew[32] found that 9.9% of patients (18/181 patients) developed a postoperative herpetic infection following dermabrasion or chemical peeling. Six percent of the patients who denied a history of herpes simplex virus (and were therefore not prophylactically treated) developed a herpetic infection. Therefore, oral antiviral prophylactic treatment is recommended following a resurfacing procedure in patients with or without a history of herpes simplex virus.

Several dosing strategies have been proposed, including acyclovir 800 mg by mouth 3 times a day, acyclovir 400 mg by mouth 3 times a day, valacyclovir 500 mg by mouth twice a day, or famciclovir 250 mg by mouth twice a day starting up to 4 days before and continuing for 2 weeks after the procedure. If a patient experiences an outbreak, a recommended treatment dose is acyclovir 800 mg 5 times a day or valacyclovir/famciclovir 500 mg 3 times a day.[10]

The use of prophylactic antibiotics is more controversial. Many laser surgeons prescribe routine antibiotics as prophylaxis against gram-positive organisms. There is no consensus on prophylactic antibiotics for laser resurfacing before an active infection is suspected.[33] Proponents of antibiotics argue that newly resurfaced skin is like a superficial burn, producing drainage and crusting that immediately becomes colonized with bacteria.[12] Thermal injury causes local immunosuppression, further predisposing the wound to infection.[34] In the past, burn units routinely administered oral prophylactic antibiotics to prevent infection, most commonly streptococcal cellulitis.[35] More recently, several studies have found that, compared with untreated controls, the use of oral prophylactic antibiotics does not decrease the incidence of infection and may increase the incidence of resistant organisms and candida colonization.[36–38] Bacterial infection risk may be decreased by acetic acid soaks and frequent occlusive dressing changes.[12] Decreasing infection risk is especially important if prophylactic antibiotics are not prescribed.

## REFERENCES

1. Black HS. Potential involvement of free radical reactions in ultraviolet light-mediated cutaneous damage. Photochem Photobiol 1987;46:213.
2. Lavker RM. Structural alterations in exposed and unexposed skin. J Invest Dermatol 1979;73:59.
3. Kligman AM. Early destructive effects of sunlight on human skin. JAMA 1969;210:2377.
4. Clark CP. Office-based skin care and superficial peels: the scientific rationale. Plast Reconstr Surg 1999;104(3):854–64.
5. Carniol PJ. Laser skin rejuvenation. Philadelphia: Lippincott-Raven; 1998.
6. Alster TS, Tanzi EL, Lazarus M. The use of fractional laser photothermolysis for the treatment of atrophic scars. Dermatol Surg 2007;33(3):295–9.
7. Koch BB, Perkins SW. Simultaneous rhytidectomy and full-face carbon dioxide laser resurfacing: a case series and meta-analysis. Arch Facial Plast Surg 2002;4(4):227–33.
8. Truswell WH IV. Combining fractional carbon-dioxide laser resurfacing with face-lift surgery. Facial Plast Surg Clin North Am 2012;20(2):201–13, vi.
9. Alster TS. Cutaneous resurfacing with CO2 and Erbium:YAG lasers: preoperative, intraoperative, and postoperative considerations. Plast Reconstr Surg 1999;103(2):619–32.
10. Alster TS, Doshi SN, Hopping SB. Combination surgical lifting with ablative laser skin resurfacing of facial skin: a retrospective analysis. Dermatol Surg 2004;30(9):1191–5.
11. Archer KA, Perkins SW. Skin resurfacing in combination with facelift surgery. Facial Plast Surg 2017; 33(3):299–310.
12. Duke D, Joop GM. Care before and after laser skin resurfacing. Dermatol Surg 2008;24:201–6.
13. Palumb A, d'Ischia M, Misuraca G. Mechanism of inhibition of melanogenesis by hydroquinone. Biochim Biophys Acta 1991;1073:85.
14. West TB, Alster TS. Effect of pretreatment on the incidence of hyperpigmentation following cutaneous CO2 laser resurfacing. Dermatol Surg 1999;25(1): 15–7.
15. Mandy SH. Tretinoin in the preoperative and postoperative management of dermabrasion. J Am Acad Dermatol 1986;15:878–9.
16. Hung VC, Lee JY, Zitelli JA, et al. Topical tretinoin and epithelial wound healing. Arch Dermatol 1989; 125:65–9.
17. Vagotis FL, Brundage SR. Histologic study of dermabrasion and chemical peel in an animal model after pretreatment with Retin-A. Aesthetic Plast Surg 1995;19:243–6.
18. Popp C, Kligman AM, Stoudemayer TJ. Pretreatment of photoaged forearm skin with topical tretinoin accelerates healing of full-thickness wounds. Br J Dermatol 1995;132:46–53.
19. Hevia O, Nemeth AJ, Taylor R. Tretinoin accelerates healing after trichloroacetic acid chemical peel. Arch Dermatol 1991;127:678–82.
20. Effendy I, Kwangsukstith C, Lee JY, et al. Functional changes in human stratum corneum induced by topical glycolic acid: comparison with all-trans retinoic acid. Acta Derm Venereol 1995;75:455–8.
21. Beasley D, Jones C, McDonald WS. Effect of pretreated skin on laser resurfacing. Laser Surg Med 1997;9(suppl):43.
22. Beach RS, Kenney MG. Vitamin A augments collagen production by corneal endothelial cells. Biochem Biophys Res Commun 1983;114: 395–402.
23. Griffiths CEM, Russman AN, Majmudar G, et al. Restoration of collagen formation of photodamaged human skin by tretinoin (retinoic acid). N Engl J Med 1993;329:530–5.
24. Kenney MC, Shih LM, Labermeier R, et al. Modulation of rabbit keratocyte production of collagen, sulfated glycosaminoglycan and fibronectin by retinol and retinoic acid. Biochim Biophys Acta 1986;889:156–62.
25. Abergel RP, Meeker CA, Oikarinen H, et al. Retinoid modulation of connective tissue metabolism in keloid fibroblast cultures. Arch Dermatol 1985;121: 632–5.
26. Jetten MA. Retinoids specifically enhance the number of epidermal growth factor receptors. Nature 1980;284:626–9.
27. Van Scott EJ, Ditre CM, Yu RJ. Alpha-hydroxyacids in the treatment of signs of photoaging. Clin Dermatol 1996;14(2):217–26.

28. DiNardo JC, Grove GL, Moy LS. Clinical and histological effects of glycolic acid at different concentrations and pH levels. Dermatol Surg 1996;22:421–4.

29. Nanni CA, Alster TS. Complications of carbon dioxide laser resurfacing: an evaluation of 500 patients. Dermatol Surg 1998;24:315.

30. Rapaport MJ, Kamer F. Exacerbation of facial herpes simplex after phenolic face peels. J Dermatol Surg Oncol 1984;10:57–8.

31. Brody HJ. Complications of chemical peeling. J Dermatol Surg Oncol 1989;15:1010–9.

32. Perkins SW, Sklarew EC. Prevention of facial herpetic infections after chemical peel and dermabrasion: new treatment strategies in the prophylaxis of patients undergoing procedures of the perioral area. Plast Reconstr Surg 1996;98:427–33.

33. Haas AF. Practical thoughts on antibiotic prophylaxis (Letter). Arch Dermatol 1998;143:1.

34. Waldorf HA, Kauvar ANB, Geronemus RG. Response to a letter to the editor. Dermatol Surg 1995;21:940–6.

35. Timmons MJ. Are systemic prophylactic antibiotics necessary for burns? Ann R Coll Surg Engl 1983; 65:80–1.

36. Krizek TJ, Gottlieb LJ, Koss N, et al. The use of prophylactic antibacterials in plastic surgery; a 1980's update. Plast Reconstr Surg 1985;76:953–63.

37. Boss WK, Brand DA, Acampora D, et al. Effectiveness of prophylactic antibiotics in the outpatient treatment of burns. J Trauma 1985;25:224–7.

38. Durtshi MB, Orgain C, counts G, et al. A prospective study of prophylactic penicillin in acutely burned hospitalized patients. J Trauma 1982;22:11–4.

# Easy Platelet-Rich Fibrin (Injectable/Topical) for Post-resurfacing and Microneedle Therapy

Richard D. Gentile, MD, MBA[a,b,*]

## KEYWORDS

• PRF • Microneedle therapy • Platelets • Platelet-rich plasma

## KEY POINTS

- The process of obtaining blood biologics, including platelet-rich plasma (PRP) and platelet-rich fibrin (PRF), can be complicated and expensive and is influenced by many vendors and proprietary techniques.
- The indications for PRP/PRF use remain controversial, and complicated or expensive modes of generating this biologic may lead to many facial plastic surgeons to pass on the use of these potentially useful agents.
- The lack of standardization of PRP procurement has also led to difficulties in assessing clinical efficacy and comparing study protocols.

## CLASSIFICATION AND HISTORY OF BLOOD-DERIVED BIOLOGICS

Platelet-rich plasma (PRP) is commonly identified as a biologic conduit for platelet-rich growth factors (GFs). In the spectrum of PRP also exists platelet-rich fibrin (PRF) matrix, PRF, and platelet concentrate. Hematologists first described the concept and content of PRP more than 40 years ago; there has always been confusion mostly related to the lack of consensual terminology, characterization, and classification of the many products that have been evaluated and tested over this time period.[1] Hematologists created the term PRP in the 1970s in order to describe the plasma with a platelet count above that of peripheral blood, which was initially used as a transfusion product to treat patients with thrombocytopenia.[2] Ten years later, PRP started to be used in maxillofacial surgery as PRF. Fibrin had the potential for adherence and homeostatic properties, and PRP, with its anti-inflammatory characteristics, stimulated cell proliferation.[3] Subsequently, PRP has been used predominantly in the musculoskeletal field in sports injuries. With its use in professional athletes, it has attracted widespread attention in the media and has been extensively used in this field.[4] Other medical fields that also use PRP are cardiac surgery, pediatric surgery, gynecology, urology, plastic surgery, and ophthalmology.[5] More recently, the interest in the application of PRP in dermatology and aesthetics, that is, in tissue regeneration, wound healing, scar revision, skin rejuvenating effects, and alopecia, has increased.[1,6–14] Wounds have a proinflammatory biochemical environment that impairs healing in chronic ulcers. In addition, it is characterized

[a] Facial Plastic Surgery, Gentile Facial Plastic Surgery and Aesthetic Laser Center, 821 Kentwood Suite C, Youngstown, OH 44512, USA; [b] Facial Plastic Surgery, Cleveland Clinic Akron General Hospital, Akron, OH, USA
* Facial Plastic Surgery, Gentile Facial Plastic Surgery and Aesthetic Laser Center, 821 Kentwood Suite C, Youngstown, OH 44512.
E-mail address: dr-gentile@msn.com

Facial Plast Surg Clin N Am 28 (2020) 127–134
https://doi.org/10.1016/j.fsc.2019.09.011

by a high protease activity, which decreases the effective GF concentration. PRP is used as an interesting alternative treatment of recalcitrant wounds because it is a source of GFs and consequently has mitogenic, angiogenic, and chemotactic properties.[12] In cosmetic dermatology, a study performed in vitro demonstrated that PRP can stimulate human dermal fibroblast proliferation and increase type I collagen synthesis.[13] Additionally, based on histologic evidence, PRP injected in human deep dermis and immediate subdermis induces soft tissue augmentation, activation of fibroblasts, and new collagen deposition as well as new blood vessels and adipose tissue formation.[14,15] Another application of PRP is the improvement of burn scars, postsurgical scars, and acne scars.[16] According to the few articles available, PRP alone or in combination with other techniques seems to improve the quality of the skin and leads to an increase in collagen and elastic fibers. In 2006, PRP has started to be considered a potential therapeutic tool for promoting hair growth and has been postulated as a new therapy for alopecia, in both androgenetic alopecia and alopecia areata. Several studies have been published that refer to the positive effect PRP has on androgenetic alopecia, although a recent meta-analysis suggested the lack of randomized controlled trials.[17] As stated by the investigators, controlled clinical trials are considered the best way to provide scientific evidence for a treatment and avoid potential bias when assessing efficacy.[18]

### Platelets and Platelet-Rich Plasma

All blood cells derive from a common pluripotent stem cell, which may differentiate into different cell lines. Each of these cell series contains precursors that can divide and mature. Platelets, also called thrombocytes, develop from the bone marrow. Platelets are nucleated, discoid cellular elements with different sizes and a density of approximately 2 μm in diameter, the smallest density of all blood cells. The physiologic count of platelets circulating in the blood stream ranges from 150,000 platelets/μL to 400,000 platelets/μL. Platelets contain several secretory granules that are crucial to platelet function. There are 3 types of granules: dense granules, alpha granules, and lysosomes. In each platelet there are approximately 50 to 80 granules, the most abundant of the 3 types of granules. Platelets are primarily responsible for the aggregation process. The main function is to contribute to homeostasis through 3 processes: adhesion, activation, and aggregation. During a vascular lesion, platelets

are activated, and their granules release factors that promote coagulation.[19] Initially they were thought to have only hemostatic activity, although, in recent years, scientific research and technology have provided a new perspective on platelets and their functions. Studies suggest that platelets contain an abundance of GFs and cytokines that can affect inflammation, angiogenesis, stem cell migration, and cell proliferation.[20] PRP is a natural source of signaling molecules, and, on activation of platelets in PRP, the Platelet-granules are degranulated and release the GFs and cytokines that modify the pericellular microenvironment. Some of the most important GFs released by platelets in PRP include vascular endothelial GF, fibroblast GF, platelet-derived GF, epidermal GF, hepatocyte GF, insulin-like GF 1, insulin-like GF 2, matrix metalloproteinases 2 and 9, and interleukin 8.[1,21]

## CLASSIFICATION OF PLATELET-RICH PLASMA AND BLOOD-DERIVED BIOLOGICS

Following the debates about the contents and the role of the various components of these preparations, a first classification was proposed in 2009[22] and is now widely cited as a milestone in the process of clarification of the terminology. This classification is simple and separates the products according to at least 2 key parameters: the presence of cell content (mostly leukocytes) and the fibrin architecture. This separation allows defining 4 main families to regroup the products.

1. Pure PRP (P-PRP)—or leukocyte-poor PRP—products are preparations without leukocytes and with a low-density fibrin network after activation. Per definition, all the products of this family can be used as liquid solutions or in an activated gel form. They can, therefore, be injected (for example, in sports medicine) or placed during gelling on a skin wound or suture (like the use of fibrin glues). Many methods of preparation exist, particularly using cell separators (continuous-flow plasmapheresis) from a hematology laboratory, as suggested by many investigators, even if this method is too heavy to be used frequently and easily in daily practice. The literature on this technique remains difficult to evaluate, because most articles were produced by the companies promoting them.[23]
2. Leukocyte-rich and PRP (L-PRP) products are preparations with leukocytes and with a low-density fibrin network after activation. Per definition, like P-PRP, all the products of this family can be used as liquid solutions or in an

activated gel form.[24] They can, therefore, be injected (for example in sports medicine) or placed during gelling on a skin wound or suture (like the use of fibrin glues). It is in this family that the largest number of commercial or experimental systems exists, with many interesting results in general surgery[25] and in orthopedic and sports medicine.[26] In particular, many automated protocols have been developed in the past 10 years, requiring the use of specific kits that allow minimum handling of the blood samples and maximum standardization of the preparations.

3. Pure PRF (P-PRF)—or leukocyte-poor PRF—products are preparations without leukocytes and with a high-density fibrin network. Per definition, these products exist only in a strongly activated gel form and cannot be injected or used like traditional fibrin glues. Because of their strong fibrin matrix, however, they can be handled like a real solid material for other applications. The main inconveniences of this technique remain its cost and relative complexity in comparison to the other forms of PRF available, the leukocyte-rich fibrin and platelet-rich fibrin (L-PRF) products.

4. L-PRF products are preparations with leukocytes and with a high-density fibrin network.[27] Per definition, these products exist only in a strongly activated gel form and cannot be injected or used like traditional fibrin glues. Because of their strong fibrin matrix, however, they can be handled like a real solid material for other applications.

## Platelet-Rich Fibrin

PRF was first developed in France by Choukroun and colleagues[28] for specific use in oral and maxillofacial surgery. Initially only the activated PRF or clotted PRF (A-PRF) was used. The PRF is a second-generation platelet concentrate, which is an improvement over traditionally prepared PRP. It is the purpose of this article to make surgeons familiar with the nonactivated injectable/topical are routes of application of iPRF, that can be used topically after skin rejuvenation procedures for treatment of alopecia or for injection, as with the Vampire (Charles E. Runels, Jr. DBA Studio Medicine, Fairhope, AL) procedures introduced in the past decade. Fibrin, which is the activated form of a plasma molecule called fibrinogen,[29] is a soluble fibrillary molecule and is massively present not only in the plasma but also in the platelet $\alpha$-granules. It plays a potential role in platelet aggregation during homeostasis, and the fibrin matrix also has the property of angiogenesis.[30,31]

Also, fibrinogen is the final substrate of all coagulation reactions. Being a soluble protein, it is transformed into an insoluble fibrin by thrombin, whereas the polymerized fibrin gel constitutes the first cicatricial matrix of the injured site.[32–34] PRF is an immune and platelet concentrate collecting on a single fibrin membrane, containing all the constituents of a blood sample that are favorable to healing and immunity.[29] This new biomaterial looks like an autologous cicatrical matrix, which is neither like fibrin glue nor like a classical platelet concentrate. It is simply centrifuged blood without any addition.[29] PRF consists of a fibrin matrix polymerized in a tetra molecular structure, with incorporation of platelets, leukocytes, cytokines, and circulating stem cells.[27,35] Clinical studies reveal that this biomaterial is a favorable matrix for the development of a coherent healing, without any inflammatory excess. PRF in the form of a platelet gel can be used in conjunction with bone grafts, which has several advantages, such as promoting wound healing, bone growth and maturation, wound sealing, and hemostasis and imparting better handling properties to graft materials.[28] It also can be used as a membrane. The topical/injectable form is more useful to core physicians and facial plastic surgeons and its protocol is discussed.

## DIFFERENCES AND SIMILARITIES BETWEEN PLATELET-RICH PLASMA AND PLATELET-RICH FIBRIN

PRF belongs to a new generation of platelet concentrate; it represents a new step in the platelet gel therapeutic concepts, with simplified processing and with no artificial biochemical modification. PRF includes cytokines, polysaccharide chains, and structural glycoproteins enmeshed within a slowly polymerized autologous fibrin network. PRF releases high quantities of 3 main GFs, transforming growth factor β1, platelet-derived GF–AB, and vascular endothelial GF, and an important coagulation matricellular glycoprotein (thrombospondin-1) for 7 days. Platelet biologics contain important GFs that increase cell proliferation, collagen production, chemotaxis, angiogenesis, and cell differentiation. PRP and PRF are concentrated platelets suspension in a small amount of plasma. Moreover, PRP and PRF contain 3 adhesive molecules (fibrin, fibronectin, and vitronectin) that play a crucial role in wound healing, particularly in extracellular matrix formation and also in epithelialization. The major difference between these 2 products is their polymerization that leads to their different biologic characteristics. Polymerization of PRP is induced by addition of anticoagulants, but PRF polymerization is a natural and slow process. Hence, PRF has more suitable fibrin network for storage of cytokines and GFs and for cell migration.[36]

## PROTOCOL FOR INJECTABLE/TOPICAL EASY PLATELET-RICH FIBRIN (KIT-FREE PRODUCTION)

When contemplating the use of PRP/PRF as a healing adjuvant after ablative or microablative skin procedures, several considerations are recognized. Because activated PRF in its original composition for use in dentistry and oral surgery is primarily as a clot, it is not as useful for topical or injectable indications in facial plastic surgery and aesthetic skin care. Its uses are far more facilitate and can be more easily applied in topical/injectable form for skin rejuvenation protocols. The composition of PRF has, in addition to the platelets, leukocytes, and stem cells, some advantages over PRP, which lacks the leukocytes and stem cells, discussed previously. One key technical point in making a kit-free PRF includes having a centrifuge capable of slow spins, including 750 rpm. The spin duration (3–5 minutes) is lower than in the PRP production of 10 minutes at 3000 rpm. A second important production technical point is that the spin preferably can be conducted in plastic tubes because there is reduced proclivity for initiating the clotting profile in plastic tubes versus glass tubes.[37] The author prefers to spin the blood draw syringes after capping the bottom, removing the plunger, and capping the top of the syringe. When spun at slow speeds in the capped plastic blood draw syringes, it is possible to draw the plasma from the plastic tubes well before the clot is formed. The obtained plasma from the plastic tubes looked like that when preparing PRP.[37] No anticoagulant agent was needed, however, to maintain the liquidity of the blood in plastic tubes spun at low spin rates. Moreover, the plasma formed a gel without adding thrombin and could glue cartilage and bone graft particles together. Instead of carrying the particulate bone piece by piece, it is possible to easily transfer the gelatinous bone particles to the recipient site as a single clump or graft. Recently, this cartilage gelling technique has become popular in performing cartilage grafts for rhinoplasty and revision rhinoplasty.

## STEPS IN PRODUCING EASY PLATELET-RICH FIBRIN FOR INJECTABLE OR TOPICAL USE

Step 1: blood draw—this is completed with an idea of how much product is needed.

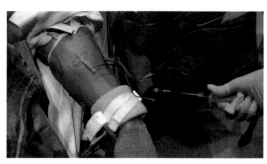

**Fig. 1.** Venipuncture and, depending on volume of PFR desired, 12-mL blood yields approximately 4-mL PRF.

Generally, 1 or 2 plastic syringes, 12 mL, are drawn after butterfly access to upper extremity venous access (**Fig. 1**).

Step 2: capping syringes—for the centrifuge spin, a lower Luer-Lock cap is placed and the plunger from the blood draw syringe is removed. The black cap is removed from plunger and used to cap the top of syringe (**Fig. 2**).

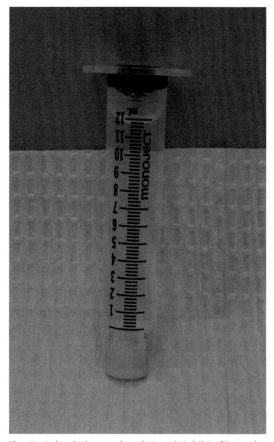

**Fig. 2.** Polyethylene tubes (12 mL) inhibit fibrin clot formation for 15 minutes to 20 minutes.

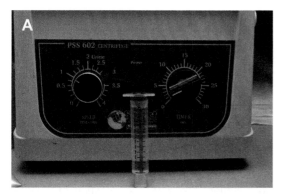
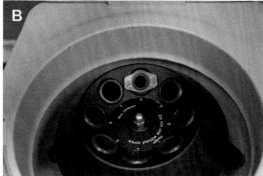

**Fig. 3.** (*A*) Centrifuge settings, 750 rpm for 3 minutes to 5 minutes; tube is capped before placement in centrifuge. (*B*) Blood draw tube placed in centrifuge; black cap from plunger used to reduce contain blood in tube.

Step 3: centrifuge spin—capped syringes are placed in the centrifuge and the centrifuge is set for 750 rpm and 3 minutes to 5 minutes (**Fig. 3**).

Step 4: remove tubes from centrifuge and place in rack remove upper cap (**Fig. 4**).

Step 5: use blunt or sharp needle on syringe to aspirate amber PRF layer (**Fig. 5**).

Step 6: use topically or inject—depending on indication. Solution is stable and does not clot for approximately 15 minutes. If using PRF to compose cartilage or bone graft, thrombin or calcium chloride can be added to promote faster activation of fibrin clot (**Fig. 6**).

## CLINICAL APPLICATION FOR PLATELET-RICH PLASMA/PLATELET-RICH FIBRIN

PRP injection has been used extensively in various clinical settings, including heart surgery, sports medicine, and wound care. PRP has attracted attention in these medical fields due to a wide variety of potential clinical benefits. Yet PRP has just recently gained increased popularity in aesthetic

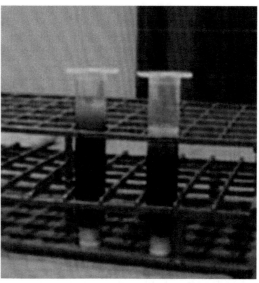

**Fig. 4.** Appearance of PRF after slow-spin intermediate layer above contains leukocytes and stem cells.

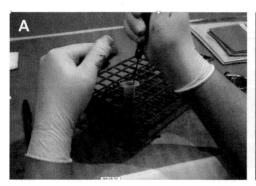
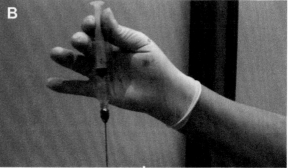

**Fig. 5.** (*A*) Using blunt-tipped needle to aspirate PRF. (*B*) Appearance of PRF without the intermediate layer.

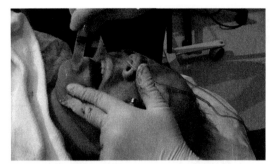

**Fig. 6.** Using PRF topically after skin rejuvenation.

surgery despite uncertainty surrounding objective clinical evidence. In PRP procedures, a small sample of the patient's own blood is processed to release various GFs from platelets—specialized blood cells involved in clotting.

In recent years, PRP injection or topical application has become a trending therapy in aesthetic medicine with increased use in core aesthetic specialties. Despite an uptick in usage, the research supporting the clinical effectiveness of these platelet biologics is limited. In a review and update, Hazen and colleagues[38] analyzed 22 published studies of PRP for specific types of facial aesthetic procedures; 14 studies evaluated the use of PRP for facial rejuvenation. All studies reported positive aesthetic outcomes with PRP injection on its own or combined with fat grafting. Reported benefits of PRP included improvements in the volume, texture, and tone of the facial skin and decreased appearance of wrinkles. Six studies using PRP to treat a specific type of hair loss called androgenic alopecia (male or female pattern baldness) reported good results in terms of hair regrowth. Androgenic alopecia is perhaps the most convincing indication for treatment with PRP, according to Hazen and colleagues.[38] Another 2 studies found positive results with the use of PRP to treat facial acne scars. Despite these encouraging results, the

review highlights several limitations of the evidence on PRP for facial aesthetic procedures. Methods of PRP preparation and injection vary considerably; some reports provided no information on the preparation technique. The studies also lacked standardized, objective assessments of skin quality before and after PRP treatment. Other issues included a lack of control (comparison) groups and follow-up to determine whether the benefits of PRP persist over time. Thus, despite many studies reporting promising results, the true value of these procedures remains open to question. "To date, the question of whether PRP's cocktail of GFs generates a more youthful appearance has not been definitively answered," the researchers write. They note that PRP injection seems safe, with a low complication rate. Hazen and coauthors emphasize the need for formal randomized, controlled trials of PRP of facial cosmetic procedures—including standardized preparation techniques, standard outcome measures, and longer follow-up. They conclude, "In the interim, this review presents a consolidation of PRP treatment techniques currently in use, to help guide physicians in their own clinical practice."

## SUMMARY

The process of obtaining blood biologics, including PRP and PRF, can be complicated and expensive and is influence by many vendors and proprietary techniques. The indications for PRP/PRF use remain controversial, and complicated or expensive modes of generating this biologic may lead to many facial plastic surgeons to pass on the use of these potentially useful agents. The lack of standardization of PRP procurement also has led to difficulties in assessing clinical efficacy and comparing study protocols. This article presents an easy protocol for producing injectable and topical PRF that is simple and inexpensive to perform. and requires no proprietary protocols or

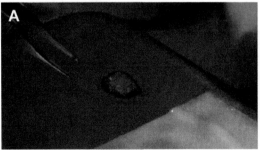
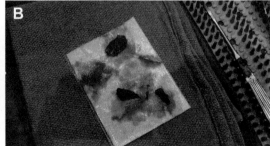

**Fig. 7.** (*A*) Using PRF for composite graft of cartilage and soft tissue. (*B*) Grafts for rhinoplasty have fibrin adhesiveness after approximately 15 minutes outside polyethylene tube.

kits. The use of a simple standard low-cost method of preparation may help standardize research protocols and permit the comparison of results from similar treatment biologics. Easy preparation may lead to more widespread use and the ability to establish clinical efficacy in various cosmetic procedures performed by core specialists. The injectable and topical formulation of PRF also can be utilized in rhinoplasty surgery to help form sticky grafts (**Fig. 7**) for rhinoplasty or revision rhinoplasty.[39]

## DISCLOSURE

None.

## REFERENCES

1. Andia I, Abate M. Platelet rich plasma: underlying biology and clinical correlates. Regen Med 2013;8: 645–58.
2. Andia I. Platelet-rich plasma biology. In: Alves R, Grimalt R, editors. Clinical indications and treatment protocols with platelet-rich plasma in dermatology. Barcelona (Spain): Ediciones Mayo; 2016. p. 3–15.
3. Conde Montero E, Fernández Santos ME, Suárez Fernández R. Platelet-rich plasma: applications in dermatology. Actas Dermosifiliogr 2015;106:104–11.
4. Lynch MD, Bashir S. Applications of plateletrich plasma in dermatology: a critical appraisal of the literature. J Dermatolog Treat 2016;27:285–9.
5. Andia E, Rubio-Azpeitia J, Martin I, et al. Current concepts and translational uses of platelet rich plasma biotechnology. In: Ekin ci D, editor. Biotechnology. London: IntechOpen Limited; 2015. https://doi.org/10.5772/59954. https://www.intechopen.com/books/biotechnology/current-concepts-and-translational-uses-of-plateletrich-plasma-biotechnology.
6. Alves R, Grimalt R. A review of platelet-rich plasma: history, biology, mechanism of action, and classification. Skin Appendage Disord 2018;4:18–24.
7. Li ZJ, Choi HI, Choi DK, et al. Autologous platelet-rich plasma: a potential therapeutic tool for promoting hair growth. Dermatol Surg 2012;38:1040–6.
8. Sommeling CE, Heyneman A, Hoeksema H, et al. The use of platelet-rich plasma in plastic surgery: a systematic review. J Plast Reconstr Aesthet Surg 2013;66:301–11.
9. Salazar-Álvarez AE, Riera-del-Moral LF, García-Arranz M, et al. Use of platelet-rich plasma in the healing of chronic ulcers of the lower extremity. Actas Dermosifiliogr 2014;105:597–604.
10. Picard F, Hersant B, Bosc R, et al. Should we use platelet-rich plasma as an adjunct therapy to treat "acute wounds", "burns", and "laser therapies": a review and a proposal of a quality criteria checklist for further studies. Wound Repair Regen 2015;23: 163–70.
11. Cobos R, Aizpuru F, Parraza N, et al. Effectiveness and efficiency of platelet rich plasma in the treatment of diabetic ulcers. Curr Pharm Biotechnol 2015;16:630–4.
12. Sclafani AP, Azzi J. Platelet preparations for use in facial rejuvenation and wound healing: a critical review of current literature. Aesthetic Plast Surg 2015;39:495–505.
13. Conde Montero E. PRP in wound healing. In: Alves R, Grimalt R, editors. Clinical indications and treatment protocols with platelet-rich plasma in dermatology. Barcelona (Spain): Ediciones Mayo; 2016. p. 59–72.
14. Kim DH, Je YJ, Kim CD, et al. Can platelet-rich plasma be used for skin rejuvenation? Evaluation of effects of platelet-rich plasma on human dermal fibroblast. Ann Dermatol 2011;23:424–31.
15. Sclafani AP, McCormick SA. Induction of dermal collagenesis, angiogenesis, and adipogenesis in human skin by injection of platelet-rich fibrin matrix. Arch Facial Plast Surg 2012;14:132–6.
16. Lola Bou Camps. PRP in cosmetic dermatology. In: Alves R, Grimalt R, editors. Clinical indications and treatment protocols with platelet-rich plasma in dermatology. Barcelona (Spain): Ediciones Mayo; 2016. p. 45–57.
17. Girão L. PRP and other applications in dermatology. In: Alves R, Grimalt R, editors. Clinical indications and treatment protocols with platelet-rich plasma in dermatology. Barcelona (Spain): Ediciones Mayo; 2016. p. 73–8.
18. Giordano S, Romeo M, Lankinen P. Plateletrich plasma for androgenetic alopecia: does it work? Evidence from meta analysis. J Cosmet Dermatol 2017;16(3):374–81.
19. Ayatollahi A, Hosseini H, Gholami J, et al. Platelet rich plasma for treatment of non-scarring hair loss: systematic review of literature. J Dermatolog Treat 2017;28(7):574–81.
20. Theml H. Physiology and pathophysiology of blood cells. In: Theml H, Diem H, Haferlach T, editors. Color atlas of hematology. Stuttgart (Germany): Thieme; 2004.
21. Harmon K, Hanson R, Bowen J, et al. Guidelines for the use of platelet rich plasma. Available at: https://www.scribd.com/document/159334949/206I CMS-Guidelines-for-the-Use-of-PlateletRich-Plasma-Draftob-oasbonasdandbowndoww. Accessed April 12, 2019.
22. Ferrando J, Fernández-Sartorio C, González de Cossío AC, et al. Tratamiento de la alopecia androgenetica con factores de crecimiento plaquetario. Mas Dermatol 2016;26:25–36.
23. Dohan Ehrenfest DM, Rasmusson L, Albrektsson T. Classification of platelet concentrates: from pure

platelet-rich plasma (P-PRP) to leucocyte- and platelet-rich fibrin (L- PRF). Trends Biotechnol 2009;27:158–67.

24. Dohan Ehrenfest DM, Bielecki T, Del Corso M, et al. Shedding light in the controversial terminology for platelet-rich products: platelet-rich plasma (PRP), plateletrich fibrin (PRF), platelet-leukocyte gel (PLG), preparation rich in growth factors (PRGF), classification and commercialism. J Biomed Mater Res A 2010;95:1280–2.

25. Everts PA, Hoffmann J, Weibrich G, et al. Differences in platelet growth factor release and leucocyte kinetics during autologous platelet gel formation. Transfus Med 2006;16:363368.

26. Everts PA, Hoogbergen MM, Weber TA, et al. Is the use of autologous platelet-rich plasma gels in gynecologic, cardiac, and general, reconstructive surgery beneficial? Curr Pharm Biotechnol 2012;13: 1163 1172.

27. Yuan T, Guo SC, Han P, et al. Applications of leukocyte- and platelet- rich plasma (L-PRP) in trauma surgery. Curr Pharm Biotechnol 2012;13:1173–84.

28. Dohan Ehrenfest DM, Del Corso M, Diss A, et al. Three-dimensional architecture and cell composition of a Choukroun's platelet-rich fibrin clot and membrane. J Periodontol 2010;81:546–55.

29. Dohan DM, Choukroun J, Diss A, et al. Platelet-rich fibrin (PRF): a second-generation platelet concentrate, Part I: Technological concepts and evolution. Oral Surg Oral Med Oral Pathol Oral Radiol Endod 2006;101:E37–44.

30. Mosesson MW, Siebenlist KR, Meh DA. The structure and biological features of fibrinogen and fibrin. Ann N Y Acad Sci 2001;936:11–30.

31. Choukroun J, Diss A, Simonpieri A, et al. Platelet-rich fibrin (PRF):A second-generation platelet concentrate, Part IV: clinical effects on tissue healing. Oral Surg Oral Med Oral Pathol Oral Radiol Endod 2006;101:E56–60.

32. Dvorak HF, Harvey VS, Estrella P, et al. Fibrin containing gels induce angiogenesis. Implications for tumor stroma generation and wound healing. Lab Invest 1987;57:673–86.

33. Clark RA. Fibrin and wound healing. Ann N Y Acad Sci 2001;936:355–67.

34. Collen A, Koolwijk P, Kroon M, et al. Influence of fibrin structure on the formation and maintenance of capillary like tubules by human microvascular endothelial cells. Angiogenesis 1998;2:153–65.

35. Van Hinsbergh VW, Collen A, Koolwijk P. Role of fibrin matrix in angiogenesis. Ann N Y Acad Sci 2001;936:426–37.

36. Choukroun J, Diss A, Simonpieri A, et al. Platelet-rich fibrin (PRF): a second-generation platelet concentrate. Part V: histologic evaluations of PRF effects on bone allograft maturation in sinus lift. Oral Surg Oral Med Oral Pathol Oral Radiol Endod 2006;101:299–303.

37. Lal Alizade F, Kazemi M, Irani S, et al. B Int J Contemp Dent Med Rev 2016;2016:030516. https://doi.org/10.15713/ins.ijcdmr.104.

38. Motosko CC, Khouri KS, Poudrier G, et al. Evaluating platelet-rich therapy for facial aesthetics and alopecia a critical review of the literature. Plast Reconstr Surg 2018;141(5):1115–23.

39. Jianpeampoolpol B, Phuminart S, Subbalekha K. Platelet-rich fibrin formation was delayed in plastic tubes. Br J Med Med Res 2016;14(9):1–9.

# Photodynamic Therapy for Photodamage, Actinic Keratosis, and Acne in the Cosmetic Practice

Lawrence S. Moy, MD*, Debra Frost, MPH, Stephanie Moy, BS

## KEYWORDS

• Photodynamic therapy • Photodamage • Acne • Intense pulsed light

## KEY POINTS

- Photodynamic Therapy has been an evolving procedure that should be very important office procedure in the use of actinic keratoses (precancerous lesions), inflammatory acne, and acne scarring.
- Photorejuvenation and skin cancer treatments are expected future treatments that will be effective with new photochemical agents and more understanding on the treatment procedure.
- Future enhancements to increase skin preparation and improve results are being studied currently. They include microneeding and chemical peels, Glycolic acid and Trichloroacetic acid, as pre treatments to increase the photochemical penetration.
- Future studies on broader wavelength spectrum light from Intense Puse LIght systems and daylight exposure are being examined for enhanced results.
- Photodynamic therapy is a simple, safe procedure with predictable efficacy in specific target skin problems and should be a possible procedure choice in most offices in facial treatments.

## INTRODUCTION

Photodynamic therapy (PDT) is the combination of the initial application of a photosensitive chemical on the skin and then using typically a blue filter light of varying spectrums afterward. As a treatment protocol, it has been more useful and functional than other chemical peels and lasers for a variety of conditions.[1] The interaction of the photosensitizing agents requires oxygen as well as the light source.[2,3] There has been efficacy in antiviral treatments, such as herpetic lesions; malignant cancers of the head and neck; and lung, bladder, and skin cancers. It has been tested for prostate cancers, cervical cancer, colorectal cancer, lung cancer, breast cancer, esophageal cancer, stomach cancer, pancreatic cancer, vaginal cancer, gliomas, and erythroplasia of Queyrat.[1,4,5]

There are 3 components required for PDT. A photosensitizer, a light source, and tissue oxygen. The wavelength of the light source is required to be within the range in nanometers to produce free radicals or reactive oxygen species.[6] These free radicals are produced by transfer from a substrate molecule, the photosensitizer, and a highly reactive state of oxygen called a singlet oxygen. The photosensitizer is applied systemically or topically to soak into the target tissue. It is then exposed to the light source for a controlled amount of time. It energizes the photosensitizer to produce the free radicals, which cause damage to the target cells, usually fast-growing cells, and at the same time with only minimal damage to the nearby healthy tissue. The photosensitizer in the excited state interacts with the molecular triplet oxygen and

Disclosures: None.
1101 North Sepulveda Boulevard, Manhattan Beach, CA 90266, USA
* Corresponding author.
E-mail address: lsm.doc@me.com

Facial Plast Surg Clin N Am 28 (2020) 135–148
https://doi.org/10.1016/j.fsc.2019.09.012

produces free radicals and reactive oxygen species. These species include singlet oxygen radicals and superoxide ions. These unstable species interact with cellular components, such as unsaturated lipids, amino acid residues, and nuclei acids. This oxidative damage results in target-cell death in the illuminated areas.[7]

In skin procedures, the application of the photosensitizer is typically topically; however, injection or oral doses can be used with certain agents. Time is needed for the agent to soak into or absorb into the target tissue. Activation of the photosensitizer requires the presence of oxygen. The combination of the photosensitizer and oxygen creates the unstable compound that, when further activated with a laser or intense pulsed light (IPL), targets hyperproliferative tissue. This treatment targets cancer or precancer cells and actinic keratoses (AKs), and preferentially spares normal surrounding tissue.[2]

## HISTORY

In the late 1800s, Finsen showed by using heat-filtered light from a carbon-arc lamp, the Finsen lamp, that phototherapy worked on lupus vulgaris, a tuberculosis condition. He won the 1903 Nobel Prize in Physiology or Medicine. Meyer-Betz, a German scientist eventually demonstrated the use of a photosensitizer by injecting himself with hematoporphyrin and then observing a general skin reaction after exposing himself to daylight sunshine.[7] Von Tappeiner and colleagues[8] performed the first PDT trial in patients with skin carcinoma using the photosensitizer, eosin. Of 6 patients with a facial basal cell carcinoma treated with a 1% eosin solution and long-term exposure either to sunlight or arc-lamp light, 4 patients showed total tumor resolution and a relapse-free period of 12 months.[9,10] One of the first dermatologic studies of the photosensitizing agents was in 1980.[7,8,11–16] Dr Patrick Abergel and Dr Jouni Uitto were working with photosensitizing agents from Kodak and interacting the agents with a neodymium:yttrium-aluminum-garnet (Nd:YAG) laser.[17,18] Initial studies showed increased collagen synthesis in fibroblasts from stimulation with the laser. Later studies examined the use of the photosensitizing agents with the blue light on surface tumors. Dougherty and coworkers[19] at Roswell Park Cancer Institute (Buffalo, NY) clinically tested PDT in 1978. They treated 113 cutaneous or subcutaneous malignant tumors with HpD and observed total or partial resolution of 111 tumors.[17] Dougherty helped expand clinical trials and formed the International Photodynamic Association in 1986. Cooper Medical Devices Corp/Cooper Lasersonics (John Toth) wrote an article on PDT with the argon dye lasers. Photofrin, a porphyria, in 1993 was the first PDT agent approved for clinical use to treat a form of bladder cancer, the first PDT treatment approved by US Food and Drug Administration (FDA) for use against certain cancers of the esophagus and non–small cell lung cancer.[7] In the 1980s, David Dolphin, Julia Levy, and colleagues[20–22] developed a novel photosensitizer, verteporfin. Verteporfin, a porphyrin derivative, is activated at 690 nm, a much longer wavelength than Photofrin. It has the property of preferential uptake by neovasculature. It has been widely tested for its use in treating skin cancers and received FDA approval in 2000 for the treatment of wet age-related macular degeneration. As such, it was the first medical treatment ever approved for this condition, which is a major cause of vision loss.

## IDEAL PHOTOSENSITIZERS

The ideal photosensitizer properly accumulates into the target tissue and biologically causes cell death to the target cells. For cutaneous use, there are several new agents that are being tested that may or may not hold up to the listed criteria.[23]

1. Strong absorption with an extended absorption at longer wavelengths in the near-visible infrared region. For example, 5-aminolevulinic acid (ALA; also known as $\delta$-aminolevulinic acid [$\delta$-ALA]) absorbs wavelengths at 400 to 410 and at 635 nm.[24]
2. Forms oxygen reactive species and free radicals readily based on the light exposures, thereby creating a reactive oxygen that leads to cytotoxicity of the target cells.
3. Low to no toxicity to the tissue before exposure to the light. Clinically stable in tissue without the light exposure.
4. Preferential penetration into the target tissue versus normal surrounding tissue. For example, goes to the hyperkeratoses of the AKs and into the pores for acne and acne scarring.
5. Rapid clearance from the body after the procedure.
6. High chemical stability.
7. Stability formulation in soluble form for clinical delivery.[25]

## PHOTOSENSITIZERS

Photosensitizers commercially available for clinical use include Allumera, Photofrin, Visudyne, Levulan, Foscan, Metvix, Hexvix, Cysview, and Laserphyrin, with others in development (eg, Antrin, Photochlor, Photosens, Photrex, Lumacan,

Cevira, Visonac, BF-200 ALA,[26,27] Amphinex,[23] and azadipyrromethenes). Porphyrin's highly conjugated skeleton produces a characteristic ultraviolet (UV)-visible (VIS) spectrum. The spectrum typically consists of an intense, narrow absorption band ($\varepsilon > 200,000$ L mol$-1$ cm$-1$) at around 400 nm, known as the Soret band or B band, followed by 4 longer-wavelength (450–700 nm), weaker absorptions ($\varepsilon > 20,000$ L·mol$-1$·cm$-1$ [free-base porphyrins]), referred to as the Q bands.[7] The Soret band arises from a strong electronic transition from the ground state to the second excited singlet state (S0 → S2), whereas the Q band is a result of a weak transition to the first excited singlet state (S0 → S1). The dissipation of energy via internal conversion is so rapid that fluorescence is only observed from depopulation of the first excited singlet state to the lower-energy ground state (S1 → S0).[7] The Soret bands at 400 nm have been the initial target for the light source. Subsequently, the Q bands from 450 to 700 nm have been targeted with some other light sources. Protoporphyrin IX (PpIX) has its largest absorption peak in the blue region at 410 nm (Soret band), with smaller absorption peaks at 505, 540, 580, and 635 nm (**Figs. 1–7**). All PpIX absorption peaks are within the visual spectrum of daylight. Disregarding tissue penetration, 87% of

the daylight PpIX activation is caused by violet-blue-cyan light (380–495 nm), whereas only 10% and 3% is activated by green-yellow (495–590 nm) and orange-red (590–750 nm) light, respectively. Most light sources for PDT seek to use the 635-nm absorption peak in the red region to improve tissue penetration. The red light penetrates more to the 2-mm range in the skin layers, which is deeper than the blue light. However, the blue light in the Soret band has a more efficient, active excitation. In the United States a blue fluorescent lamp (peak emission 417 nm) is routinely used for ALA-PDT of nonhyperkeratotic AK. Studies show that blue, green, and red light are all effective when using topical PDT to treat AK, but the deeper penetrating red light is superior when treating Bowen disease and basal cell carcinomas.[12,28]

## PHOTOSENSITIZERS

ALA,[30] an endogenous nonproteinogenic amino acid, is the first compound in the porphyrin synthesis pathway, the pathway that leads to heme[24,29] in mammals and chlorophyll[7] in plants. Based on the size and structure of the compound, it penetrates the membrane bilayer of the cells readily. The heme molecule is

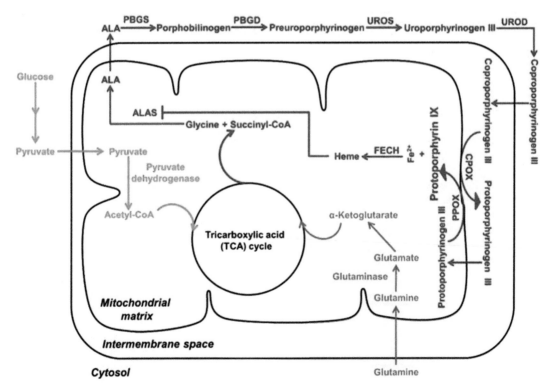

**Fig. 1.** In mitochondria, ALA and methyl-5-aminolaevulinate (MAL) are metabolites of hemoglobin breakdown and the tricarboxylic acid cycle.

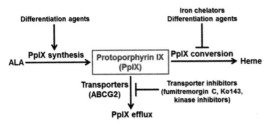

**Fig. 2.** Precursor of protoporphyria. Accumulation of porphyria compounds leads to photosensitive diseases.

synthesized from glycine and succinyl coenzyme A (succinyl CoA). The rate-limiting step in the biosynthesis pathway is controlled by a tight (negative) feedback mechanism in which the concentration of heme regulates the production of ALA. However, this controlled feedback can be bypassed by artificially adding excess exogenous ALA to cells. The cells respond by producing PpIX (photosensitizer) at a faster rate than the ferrochelatase enzyme can convert it to heme.[7] ALA, marketed as Levulan (DUSA Pharmaceuticals, Inc., Wilmington, MA), has shown promise in PDT (tumors) via both intravenous and oral administration, as well as through topical administration in the treatment of malignant and nonmalignant dermatologic conditions, including psoriasis, Bowen disease, and hirsutism (phase II/III clinical trials).[7,31] ALA accumulates more rapidly compared with other intravenously administered sensitizers. Typical peak tumor accumulation levels postadministration for PpIX are usually achieved within several hours; other (intravenous) photosensitizers may take up to 96 hours to reach peak levels. ALA is also excreted more rapidly from the body (about 24 hours) than other photosensitizers, minimizing photosensitivity side effects.[32,33] ALA has absorption wavelengths of 400 to 410 and 635 nm. ALA is available as a 20% solution .[31,34] It is FDA approved since 1999 and approved for the treatment of nonhyperkeratotic

AKs on the face and scalp in conjunction with a blue light source.[10] It is supplied as a cardboard tube housing 2 sealed glass ampules, 1 containing 354 mg of ALA hydrochloride powder and the other 1.5 mL of solvent. These separate components are mixed within the cardboard sleeve just before use.[28,35]

## Methyl-5-aminolaevulinate

Esterified ALA derivatives with improved bioavailability have been examined. A methyl ALA ester (Metvix) is now available for basal cell carcinoma and other skin lesions.[31] Benzyl (Benvix) and hexyl ester (Hexvix) derivatives are used for gastrointestinal cancers and for the diagnosis of bladder cancer.[7] An alternative to ALA is the methyl ester form, methyl-5-aminolaevulinate (MAL).[7] The presence of methyl ester group makes the molecule more lipophilic and enhances penetration; however, MAL must be demethylated back to ALA by intracellular enzymes. MAL has been shown to reach maximal intracellular concentrations of PpIX quickly, allowing a shorter incubation period. In the Unites States, MAL was available for a brief period as a 16.8% cream and marketed under the trade name Metvixia (Galderma Laboratories, LP, Fort Worth, TX). However, it is currently unavailable in the US market. In the mitochondria, ALA and MAL are metabolites of hemoglobin breakdown and the tricarboxylic acid cycle. Both of these photosensitizers are precursors of protoporphyria. As is known from several porphyria conditions, there are photosensitive diseases in which photosensitizers with sunlight cause severe sun conditions.

The porphyria compounds used in PDT are excited to a higher-energy triplet state, which either emits light (as fluorescence) or generates a reactive oxygen species, either a singlet oxygen or free radicals. The singlet oxygen does not travel far and causes molecular effects, primarily

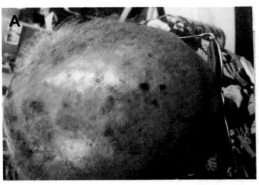
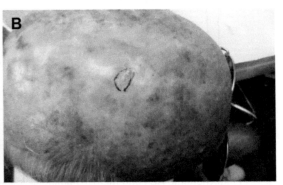

**Fig. 3.** (*A*) Before and (*B*) after ALA (Levallan) and IPL.

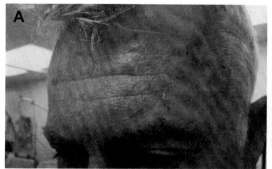
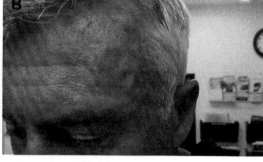

**Fig. 4.** (*A*) Before and (*B*) after ALA (Levallan) with IPL.

apoptosis or necrosis of malignant cells in the very localized area of the photosensitizer exposed to light.

## Allumera

Hexyl aminolevulinate (HAL) is an ester of ALA that has shown cosmetic benefits and minimal side effects when used in combination with red or blue light in adults with visible signs of aging and photodamage. Allumera was initially approved for use by the FDA in a thorough study of 120 patients. This double-blind controlled study used Allumera and red light treatment. The cosmetic results were: (1) revitalized, younger-looking, clearer, and more beautiful skin; (2) reduced appearance of crow's feet, dark circles, fine lines' and wrinkles; (3) firmer appearance of the skin; (4) improvement in the

feeling of moisture, smoothness, and overall skin texture. PDT with HAL and IPL improved cosmetic appearance and was generally well tolerated. PDT with a HAL-containing cosmetic cream and IPL improved cosmetic appearance (investigator and subject rated) and was generally well tolerated.[36] Overall, minimal erythema, dryness, bruising, and stinging/burning were observed. Only 1 subject experienced an adverse event (crusts following the first and second treatments, which resolved without intervention before the third treatment). These findings suggest that the combination of a HAL-containing cosmetic cream and IPL may be a useful, noninvasive, and well-tolerated cosmetic option for individuals seeking the restoration of a more youthful appearance.[37,38] Allumera is an ideal intervention for individuals who want a

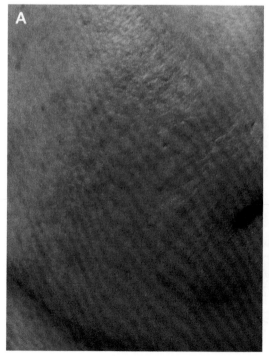
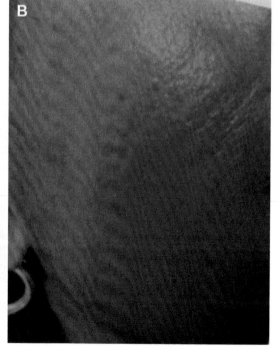

**Fig. 5.** (*A*) Before and (*B*) after Allumera with IPL.

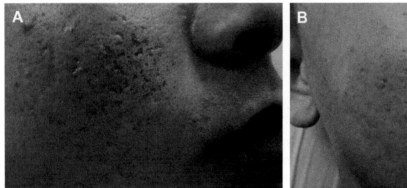
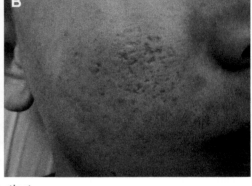

**Fig. 6.** (*A*) Before and (*B*) after Allumera with IPL in male patient.

rejuvenation procedure that provides a more dramatic improvement than a superficial chemical peel but who are not ready for a more invasive procedure. PDT successfully addresses pore size, pigmentation irregularities, texture, tone, and to some degree fine lines and wrinkles.[36]

## LIGHT SOURCE

The Blu-U light apparatus by DUSA, the same company that provides Levulan Kerastick 20% ALA, focuses on the Soret absorbance band. Its maximum wavelength output is at 417 nm. This unit is designed to have the patient enclosed in a wraparound light delivery system. The light is incoherent and nonfocused. The wraparound allows the patients to be exposed across the whole face the whole time all at once. The patient sits in the unit, as designed by DUSA, for an exposure of 16 minutes and 40 seconds.[34,39] The extended length of time helps improve the depth of the blue light penetration to hit the levels of the absorbed photosensitizers, especially the ALA. Because the typical treatment is for AKs, the target is primarily all epidermal, which means the treatment focuses on the surface effect. For rejuvenation and acne, there are some other, deeper effects in which dermal light absorbance may be more beneficial.

### Intense Pulsed Light

IPL is also incoherent, nonfocused light. The advantage of the IPL system is that it is broad spectrum of wavelengths from 400 to 1200 nm depending on the system used. The wavelengths are focused on by the variations of peaks with a choice of filters. Some increase the wavelengths that are closer to visible light and some that are in the longer, infrared region. The filters are used to center on the wide variety of targets of for IPL. The systems are used for hair removal, pigmentation, vascular lesions, rosacea, and rejuvenation. With PDT, the IPL can target the Soret band and the Q bands to get both levels of photosensitizer absorbance.[35,40]

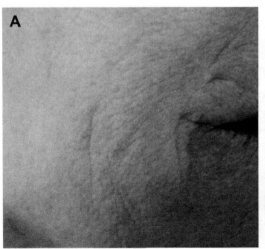
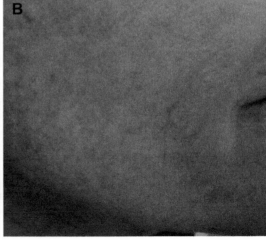

**Fig. 7.** (*A*) Before and (*B*) after ALA (Levallan) with IPL.

## Laser Systems

Lasers have been used in place of the blue light and IPL to maximize the depth of the light source for photosensitizer excitation. A ruby laser at 694 nm wavelength has a deeper penetration than an argon laser with a shorter wavelength of 488 nm. Potentially, it targets the red spectrum for the photosensitizer and targets deeper tissues. Tunable argon dye lasers, copper vapor lasers, pulse dye lasers, Nd:YAG potassium titanyl phosphate lasers, diode lasers, and gold vapor lasers have reportedly been used in PDT.[41–45]

There are several articles that have discussed PDT using the daylight spectrum to provide the light source. Hovenic and colleagues[46] showed that the use of daylight after application of the photosensitizing agent is effective and well tolerated. Two Asian studies, 1 in Korea and 1 in Japan,[47] both outlined mild to minimal side effects with acceptable tolerability and effectiveness for acne using ambient daylight exposure.[48] One study compared the amount of energy at 56° latitude with the typical photodynamic light exposure in the office. Using 30 minutes of exposure on a typically sunny day was equivalent to the office exposure with a blue light. The advantages of the daylight treatments are less pain and greater convenience of avoiding a laser or IPL procedure. Daylight is the combination of direct and diffuse sunlight outdoors during the daytime. The spectrum of electromagnetic radiation striking the Earth's atmosphere is the ultraviolet light ranging from 100 to 380 nm, visible light ranging from 380 to 780 nm, and infrared light ranging from 780 to 106 nm. During 2 hours of daylight exposure, the minimum mean illuminance should be 100,000 lux to achieve the same PpIX-weighted effective red light dose as obtained by illumination with the conventional light-emitting diode (LED) lamp used with MAL. If all wavelengths within the absorption spectrum of PpIX were equally effective in the activation of PpIX, daylight illumination for 2 hours with as little as 2300 lux would be enough to achieve the same effective light dose as is achieved with the red LED lamps. The efficacy of daylight-PDT in the treatment of multiple AKs in the face and scalp has been studied in 3 randomized clinical trials performed in Northern Europe.

In 1 study, patients were treated in a split-site design with bright sunlight–mediated PDT versus conventional red LED–mediated PDT.[49] One area was exposed to sunlight for 2.5 h in the hospital garden after half an hour of MAL under occlusion. The other area was illuminated with red LED light (37 J/ cm$^2$) 3 hours after MAL application under occlusion. Sunlight-mediated PDT was as effective as in-office PDT with a 3-month lesion response rate of 79% in the sunlight-mediated PDT area compared with 71% in the LED-PDT–treated area. PpIX fluorescence increased steadily during the 3 hours of occlusive treatment in the LED areas, whereas very little accumulation of PpIX was seen in the sunlight-treated areas. The lack of accumulation of PpIX during sunlight exposure shows that daylight exposure was sufficient to activate PpIX during its formation.

After application of a sun protection factor (SPF) 20 sunscreen on sun-exposed skin areas, including the treatment area, patients were treated with 16% and 8% MAL-PDT in 2 symmetric areas in the face and scalp. Immediately after application of the MAL cream, patients went home with instructions to spend the remaining day outside in daylight and wash off the creams before bedtime. Daylight-PDT was efficient in a home-based setting with a mean response rate of all lesion grades in the 2 treatment areas of 78.2% at the 3-month follow-up. No difference in response rates was found between areas treated with the conventional 16% MAL cream and the 8% cream ($P = .37$).[49]

In a multicenter study, after preparation with application of a sunscreen and MAL, patients left the clinic and exposed themselves to daylight according to the randomization. Patients were advised to start light exposure within 30 minutes after drug application and were instructed to wash the treatment area after daylight exposure. The mean lesion complete response rate was 76.5% at 3-month follow-up and no significant difference in response rate was found between the 1.5-hour and 2.5-hour exposure groups. This study showed that daylight-PDT is an alternative to conventional PDT for AKs, with the added convenience of being an almost pain-free therapy.[50,51]

Daylight-mediated PDT is a simpler and more tolerable treatment procedure for PDT. Three randomized controlled studies have shown that daylight-mediated PDT is an effective treatment of thin AKs.[52] Daylight-mediated PDT is nearly pain free and more convenient for both clinicians and patients. Daylight-mediated PDT is especially suited for patients with large field-cancerized areas, which can easily be exposed to daylight. Further investigations are necessary to determine at which time of the year and in which weather conditions daylight-mediated PDT is possible in different geographic locations. It is recommended to wear sunscreens on the sun-exposed areas of the skin. There can be significant pain if there is too much sun exposure as well as crusting and significant erythema. The problem with daylight PDT is that there is a variable amount of time that should be used to provide the sunlight light source.[53,54] At this time, the variables that change the light exposure have to do with the seasonal time period, the geographic area, and the latitude. More information needs to be worked out on what is the minimal amount of sunlight that is effective for daylight PDT.[55]

Light sources can vary depending on the advantages and disadvantages of each system. Our office has been using an IPL system primarily. It has the advantages of treating a large surface area with the handpiece, being able to pulse the light on the 2 wavelength peaks of ALA, and treating a wider spectrum of wavelengths. The other agents used are blue light (Blu-U, Clearlight) and red light (Aktilite, Curelight).

Other research has been focused on using PDT for the treatment of a variety of infections, including Lassa fever, Pseudomonas aeruginosa, malaria, chromoblastomycosis, Borrelia burgdorfei, Salmonella enterica, verruca, epidermodysplasia verruciformis, and human papilloma virus. Using PDT has strong antimicrobial effects and boosts the local immune cells to fight the local infection.[56–63]

Dentistry has been using PDT for dental plaques, gum disease, and dental stomatitis.

Dermatology has been focusing on use for chronic skin ulcers, onychomycosis, hidradenitis suppurativa, tinea versicolor, malassezia folliculitis, Trichophyton rubrum, tinea cruris and tinea pedis, cutaneous leishmaniasis, infected leg ulcers, and cutaneous T-cell lymphoma (mycosis fundgoides).

## Actinic Keratoses

AKs are erythematous, scaly lesions in a sun-damage skin area. These lesions are considered to be precancerous for squamous cell carcinomas. Studies have shown that the cells are altered from sun exposure to be similar to cells that form squamous cell carcinoma. These lesions are very common among the older population in certain states, such as Florida. AKs are common (estimated prevalence of 39.5 million in 2004, 26 million of which were in patients >65 years of age) epidermal lesions that have the potential to progress to invasive squamous cell carcinoma, with the highest incidence in the aged population. Chronic exposure to ultraviolet radiation in fair-skinned patients is the most important risk factor for the development of AKs. Clinically, they can vary from small erythematous scaly macules to pigmented rough patches to hyperkeratotic cutaneous horns in sun-exposed areas.[1] They are the second most common diagnosis made by dermatologists in their practices

and account for more than 5.2 million office visits a year, leading to more than $920 million spent on treatments[2,4] (https://www.ncbi.nlm.nih.gov/pmc/articles/PMC3549675/).

Clinical presentation is for the scaling to be abnormal and uneven, with the inflammation in the vicinity but just beyond the scaling. Recognition of the AKs sometimes is by feel with clinical observation. Treatments of AKs typically begin with liquid nitrogen, applied by spraying from a pressurized can or application with a cotton swab. Treatment with liquid nitrogen with a swab or with a spray can is variably effective depending on the length of time of the treatment of each lesion. Short times less than 5 seconds are about 39% effective and more than 20 seconds is 83% effective.[64–66] The limitations of liquid nitrogen are pain, blistering, hypopigmentation, hyperpigmentation, scarring, and infection.[67]

For treatment in a greater surface area or field directed area, there are several creams. Topical 5-fluourouracil is most widely used and is applied twice-daily for 6 weeks. T It causes crusting, pain, and discomfort for 8 weeks in a typical treatment. Other topical creams are imiquimod (Aldara), ingenol mebutate (Picato), and topical diclofenac sodium 3% gel. The topical creams are chosen to treat a larger area than the liquid nitrogen and can treat areas with subclinical AKs that cannot be seen.[68–71] The problems can be that there may be much more subclinical AK than clinical AK. Often new lesions appear that are not recurrent lesions that did not clear from liquid nitrogen but are subclinical lesions that never cleared. Both subclinical and clinical AKs can develop into squamous cell carcinoma; therefore, it is worth treating for both types of lesions.

Approved for lesion-directed therapy in 1999, PDT involves applying ALA or methyl 5-aminolevulinate topically, which undergo conversion to the photosensitizer PpIX in abnormal keratinocytes. Free radicals are produced after light activation, which results in targeted tissue destruction.[72] It is used off label for field therapy. Pretreatment with dermabrasion, curettage, or urea cream can increase efficacy. FDA-approved regimens include using 20% ALA solution and blue light for 16 minutes and 40 seconds or 16.8% methyl 5-aminolevulinate with red light for 7 to 10 minutes.[72]

PDT has been successfully used for AKs because of advantages compared with previous treatments. PDT treats subclinical AKs and decreases the number of subsequent AKs that can arise later, which is similar to the topical creams. However, PDT has a much shorter healing time than 5-fluourouracil, with healing in about 1 to

2 weeks. The other big advantage of PDT is the rejuvenation benefits on the other aging effects of sun damage (wrinkles, brown spots, rough texture, and sagging).[73,74]

PDT uses a light-sensitizing compound that preferentially accumulates in AK cells, where it can be activated by the appropriate wavelength of light. ALA is a component of the heme biosynthetic pathway that accumulates preferentially in dysplastic cells. Once inside these cells, it is enzymatically converted to PpIX, a potent photosensitizer. With exposure to light of an appropriate wavelength, oxygen free radicals are generated and cell death results[75] (https://emedicine.medscape.com/article/1099775-treatment). Patients experience pain, similar in scope to the pain resulting from topical 5-fluourouracil, in the areas treated. The treated lesions may become erythematous and crusted. One treatment with PDT seems to be as effective as topical 5-fluourouracil therapy.[76] A recent meta-analysis and systematic review assessed the effectiveness of PDT versus cryotherapy and found that PDT had a 14% better chance of complete lesion clearance at 3 months for thin AKs on the face and scalp compared with cryotherapy.[77] Immunosuppressed patients may also benefit from PDT in the prevention of nonmelanoma skin cancers[78] When used with light sources that have a cosmetic benefit by themselves, such as the pulsed dye laser or IPL devices, a cosmetic benefit may be seen from the use of topical PDT beyond that of AK eradication. Compared with other destructive therapeutic options, such as cryotherapy, PDT may offer better cosmetic results and higher patient preference.[78,79] An unknown parameter in the use of topical PDT is the optimal incubation time following application of the topical ALA before light exposure. A second unknown parameter is the optimal light source to use for this treatment. Ongoing studies are addressing these issues.[78,80]

Another photosensitizing agent approved in the use of PDT is MAL. Comparison studies between ALA and MAL are not currently decisive. A study investigating the clinical efficacy of ALA-PDT versus MAL-PDT in the treatment of AK, Bowen disease, nodular basal cell carcinoma, and superficial basal cell carcinoma found that there were no statistically significant differences in their treatment outcomes using either of these agents.[81] However, a randomized, multicenter, observer-blind, placebo-controlled trial comparing the efficacy of BF-200 ALA versus MAL cream in the treatment of AK lesions showed that PDT with BF-200 ALA was superior to the MAL cream regarding patient complete clearance of lesions. Six-month and 12-month follow-up studies substantiated the efficacy of PDT with BF-200 ALA and the lower recurrence rates of lesions with BF-200 ALA treatment versus MAL treatment.[82,83] Looking beyond lesion clearance, MAL-PDT was found to be less painful than ALA-PDT in a retrospective monocentric study of 173 patients.[84]

Variations of treatment or off-label variations are used at times. Incubation times can vary from 30 to 90 minutes, which can affect the depth of the photosensitizer penetration. Also, other light sources are being used, including a pulse dye laser. Treatments of basal cell carcinomas, Bowen cancer, and squamous cell carcinoma in situ are also being examined.

The patient selection is important. The authors chose the patient for AKs based on clinical recalcitrance to the liquid nitrogen treatment. Often there are stubborn or difficult lesions of the AKs and they do not resolve after multiple treatments. In addition, some patients, based on accumulated sun damage from years ago, continue to develop new AKs even with current sun protection. Typically, liquid nitrogen follow-up is 6 months. The authors have patients return from 6 weeks to 3 months when the skin is resistant to improvement in the AKs. Even with more frequent treatments, if the liquid nitrogen treatment is not adequate, then we consider and consult with the patient for PDT.

## Acne

Acne has been successfully treated with PDT. Typical acne treatments have been combined topical treatments. Retinoic acid with a topical antibiotic have conventionally been used.[85] The retinoic acid is used to eliminate the cell accumulation that blocks the pores and the topical antibiotic keeps the bacteria count in the pore down to decrease the oil breakdown that leads to inflammation.[86] At our facilities, we use glycolic acid, which works most directly on the comedomes compared with other topical agents. Glycolic acid breaks up desmosomes. Desmosomes hold the epidermal-type cells together and causes the plug that accumulates and blocks the pores.[87,88] Glycolic acid opens the pores by separating these plugs. Used with a topical antibiotic, the antibiotic penetrates deeper in the pore to decrease the bacteria count and reduce inflammation. Oral antibiotics are used also to decrease the inflammatory response and the swelling and redness that develop in highly inflammatory acne.[89,90] Glycolic acid also works on rejuvenation and stimulation of the collagen, which is effective for acne scarring.[91,92]

The PDT is effective in acne by [other slides].

For acne treatments the authors identify patients with noticeable acne scarring and/or highly inflammatory acne. Because the PDT seems to decrease cytokines reaction and reduce the bacteria counts, the inflammatory component of acne can be dramatically decreased with several treatments of PDT.[93–95] The authors have had significant success with some types of acne scarring as well. This experience corroborates studies that have been done previously.[96–98] The pore-shaped acne scars that have been difficult to treat with other chemical peels, surgery, or injections seem to be improved consistently with PDT. In these pock-marked or pore-shaped acne scars, it may be easier for the photosensitizer to penetrate into the deeper layers of the dermis. There is therefore more collagen remodeling that functionally occurs than with other treatment modalities. It is probable that pock-marked scars have most of the extensive scarring at the bottom of the pore scar.

Acne is one of the key conditions that PDT is effective for. The benefit is in allowing the photosensitizer to penetrate into the follicles. The improvements are in the inflammatory acne and in acne scarring.[99,100] Targeting sebaceous glands, the PDT heats and ablates the sebaceous gland activity. There is also an antibacterial effect on the acne that targets propionibacterium acne and breaks up the bacteria biofilm.[101,102] In addition, there is selective immune cell necrosis that dampens or decreases the inflammatory response. Over time, the authors suspect that there is an arrest of follicular hyperkeratosis, thereby decreasing future plugging and follicular occlusion.

Acne inflammatory responses seem to be responsible for the difficulty in controlling acne exacerbations and lead to more permanent scarring. Inhibition of cytokines responses is considered to be a major factor in the benefits of PDT. The cytokines with inhibition include interleukin 1, interleukin 2, tumor necrosis factor alpha, granulocyte monocyte colony-stimulating factor , interleukin 8, interleukin 1-beta, matrix metalloproteinase-9, and phosphorylase nuclear factor-kappa B.

There have been studies to prove that collagen remodeling, and hence skin rejuvenation, results from PDT. There are some photosensitizers that diffuse into the papillary dermis and, as mentioned earlier, deeper into the reticular dermis layers in the pores. Increased collagen deposition has been noted in histologic studies.

## PROCEDURE
### Actinic Keratoses: Face

In the treatment of AKs, the authors always explain that there will be 2 treatments within 5 weeks apart. The 2 treatments are designed to provide the standard time for the photosensitizer application 3 times evenly with the blue IPL source to the required areas. Two days after the first treatment session, we evaluate the patient's response and alter the second treatment based on the amount of erythema and crusting. This ensures that there is a sufficient response to clear the AKs.

Cleansing is performed with alcohol and acetone. As with chemical peels, it is important to strip the stratum corneum and surface epidermal oils evenly. It is critical to keep the cleansing consistent and uniform. Other agents may be used, but the alcohol and acetone are more consistent at lifting off the top keratinizing layer.

The photosensitizer is applied liberally and evenly, massaging it in more vigorously to the areas with more involved AKs. The 20% ALA is our standard photosensitizer for AKs. The areas are rubbed in enough that the area is kept moist at first. The patient is then allowed to sit for 1.5 hours for the first session.

Typically, the authors use the blue light filter for the Alma Soprano with the 420-nm to 950-nm filter. The settings are constant with an 8-J single pulse at 30 microseconds. The area is treated 3 times evenly to cover the whole face. Difficult localized areas of AKs are treated 4 or 5 times. Immediately after the treatment, we apply a mild cortisone cream, and sunscreen. The patient is instructed to wear a hat if walking to the car and driving. The patient must stay indoors for 48 hours. After 48 hours, SPF 30 sunscreen and other protections such as a hat and umbrella should be used for the following 3 days.

At 2 days, we evaluate the patient very carefully. We assess the patient response based on reactions, such as the amount of redness, crusting, and scaling present. A photograph is taken and, based on the reaction at 2 days, it is then determined how strong the second treatment will be. Gauging the patient's response allows us to increase the effectiveness of the second treatment. During the second treatment, we leave the photosensitizer on the skin for up to 2 hours, and longer if we require more reaction and therefore more penetration of the photosensitizer. The light source is on the same settings. We maintain the same filter of 420 to 950 nm with the same settings of 8 J and single pulse at 30 microseconds.

Healing after treatment of AKs consistently involves 1 full week of erythema. Typically there is little to no crusting. With the acne treatments, there is typically 5 days of erythema. There is a 30% chance of hyperpigmentation within the first

6 weeks. Mild 4% hydroquinone lightens the skin pigmentation quickly, within 1 month. With both treatments, sun protection is very important to reduce the pigmentation load within the first 6 weeks. Patient preparation requires instructing patients to minimize sun exposure 2 weeks before and 4 weeks after the procedure. During the application of the photosensitizer, and 1 week later, no sun exposure is mandatory, except if the patient is doing PDT with daylight treatment exposure.

### Actinic Keratoses: Chest, Legs, Back

The procedure is the same as for the face. The Levulan is applied for 3 to 4 hours, which is longer than on the face. Again, we have the patient return in 2 days to evaluate the response to modify the second treatment.

### Acne Face

The authors use Allumera for acne and acne scarring. It can also be used for rejuvenation. It has the ability to work between light chemical peels and stronger laser resurfacing. As a combination product procedure, patients understand that explanation.[36]

The authors use 2 photosensitizers. Both are ALA. As mentioned, we use the 20%, Levulan Kerastick, for AKs and photorejuvenation. We use 4% ALA for acne and acne scarring.

### In the Future

Various improvements that are being investigated for the future. Our office is planning studies with microneedling to prep the skin and increase the photosensitizer skin penetration as part of the preparation step. Other chemical peels, including tricholoacetic acid or glycolic acid, are being considered to improve the photosensitizer penetration. In addition, other photosensitizers are being studied for future use in dermatology. Some other porphyria compounds are being examined for use in specific target areas. Skin cancers and photorejuvenation are also being examined more closely to expand the types of treatments that PDT can be effective for. Different chemical variations of ALA are being investigated in several studies.

## REFERENCES

1. Saini R, Lee NV, Liu KY, et al. Prospects in the application of photodynamic therapy in oral cancer and premalignant lesions. Cancers (Basel) 2016; 8(9) [pii:83].

2. Wang SS, Chen J, Keltner L, et al. New technology for deep light distribution in tissue for phototherapy. Cancer J 2002;8(2):154–63.

3. Lane N. New light on medicine. Scientific American; 2003.

4. Swartling J, Höglund OV, Hansson K, et al. Online dosimetry for temoporfin-mediated interstitial photodynamic therapy using the canine prostate as model. J Biomed Opt 2016;21(2):028002.

5. Swartling J, Axelsson J, Ahlgren G, et al. System for interstitial photodynamic therapy with online dosimetry: first clinical experiences of prostate cancer. J Biomed Opt 2010;15(5):058003.

6. Skovsen E, Snyder JW, Lambert JD, et al. Lifetime and diffusion of singlet oxygen in a cell. J Phys Chem B 2005;109(18):8570–3.

7. Josefsen LB, Boyle RW. Photodynamic therapy and the development of metal-based photosensitisers. Met Based Drugs 2008;2008:276109.

8. Raab O. Über die Wirkung Fluorescierenden Stoffe auf Infusorien. Z Biol 1904;39:524–46.

9. von Tappeiner H, Jesionek H. Therapeutische Versuche mit fluoreszierenden Stoffen. MMW Munch Med Wochenschr 1903;50:2042–4.

10. Jesionek H, von Tappeiner H. Zur Behandlung der Hautcarcinome mit fluoreszierenden Stoffen. Dtsch Arch Klin Med 1905;82:223–6.

11. von Tappeiner H, Jodlbauer A. Über die Wirkung der photodynamischen (fluorescierenden) Stoffe auf Protozoen und Enzyme. Dtsch Arch Klin Med 1904;80:427–87.

12. Policard A. Etudes sur les aspects offerts par des tumeurs experimentales examines a la lumiere de Wood. C R Seances Soc Biol Fil 1924;91: 1423–4.

13. Figge FH, Weiland GS, O Manganiello L. Studies on cancer detection and therapy; the affinity of neoplastic, embryonic, and traumatized tissue for porphyrins, metalloporphyrins, and radioactive zinc hematoporphyrin. Anat Rec 1948;101:657.

14. Lipson RL, Baldes EJ. The photodynamic properties of a particular hematoporphyrin derivative. Arch Dermatol 1960;82(4):508–16.

15. Lipson RL, Baldes EJ, Olsen AM. The use of a derivative of hematoporhyrin in tumor detection. J Natl Cancer Inst 1961;26:1–11.

16. Lipson RL, Baldes EJ, Gray MJ. Hematoporphyrin derivative for detection and management of cancer. Cancer 1967;20(12):2255–7.

17. Castro DJ, Abergel RP, Meeker C, et al. Effects of the Nd:YAG laser on DNA synthesis and collagen production in human skin fibroblast cultures. Ann Plast Surg 1983;11(3):214–22.

18. Castro DJ, Abergel RP, Johnston KJ, et al. Wound healing: biological effects of Nd:YAG laser on collagen metabolism in pig skin in comparison to thermal burn. Ann Plast Surg 1983;11(2):131–40.

19. Moan J, Peng Q. An outline of the history of PDT. In: Thierry patrice. Photodynamic therapy. Comprehensive series in photochemistry and photobiology, vol. 2. The Royal Society of Chemistry; 2003. p. 1–18.

20. Richter A, Sternberg E, Waterfield E, et al. Characterization of benzoporphyrin derivative a new photosensitizer. Proc SPIE Int Soc Opt Eng 1990; 997:145–50.

21. Richter A, Waterfield E, Jain AK, et al. Photosensitizing potency of benzoporphyrin derivative (BPD) in a mouse tumor model. Photochem Photobiol 1990;52(3):495–500.

22. Wilson BC, Patterson MS. The physics, biophysics, and technology of photodynamic therapy. Phys Med Biol 2008;53(9):R61–109.

23. O'Connor AE, Gallagher WM, Byrne AT. Porphyrin and nonporphyrin photosensitizers in oncology: preclinical and clinical advances in photodynamic therapy. Photochem Photobiol 2009;85(5): 1053–74.

24. Malik Z, Djaldetti M. 5 aminolevulinic acid stimulation of porphyrin and hemoglobin synthesis by uninduced Friend erythroleukemic cells. Cell Differ 1979;8(3):223–33.

25. Lee TK, Baron ED, Foster THH. Monitoring Pc 4 photodynamic therapy in clinical trials of cutaneous T-cell lymphoma using noninvasive spectroscopy. J Biomed Opt 2008;13(3):030507.

26. Allison RR, Downie GH, Cuenca R, et al. Photosensitizers in clinical PDT. Photodiagnosis Photodyn Ther 2004;1(1):27–42.

27. Huang Z. A review of progress in clinical photodynamic therapy. Technol Cancer Res Treat 2005; 4(3):283–93.

28. Morton CA, Brown SB, Collins S, et al. Guidelines for topical photodynamic therapy: report of a workshop of the British Photodermatology Group. Br J Dermatol 2002;146:552–67.

29. Gardener LC, Cox TM. Biosynthesis of heme in immature erythroid cells. J Biol Chem 1988;263: 6676–82.

30. Wettstein D, Gough S, Kannangara CG. Chlorophyll biosynthesis. Plant Cell 1995;7:1039–57.

31. Babilas P, Schreml S, Landthaler M, et al. Photodynamic therapy in dermatology: state-of-the-art. Photodermatol Photoimmunol Photomed 2010;26: 118–32.

32. Van der veen N, De bruijn HS, Berg RJ, et al. Kinetics and localisation of PpIX fluorescence after topical and systemic ALA application, observed in skin and skin tumours of UVB-treated mice. Br J Cancer 1996;73:925–30.

33. Golub AL, Gudgin dickson EF, Kennedy JC, et al. The monitoring of ALA-induced protoporphyrin IX accumulation and clearance in patients with skin lesions by in vivo surface-detected fluorescence spectroscopy. Lasers Med Sci 1999;14:112–22.

34. Goldman MP, Fitzpatrick RE, Ross EV, et al. Lasers and energy devices for the skin. Boca Raton (FL): CRC Press; 2013.

35. Star WM, Aalders MC, Sac A, et al. Quantitative model calculation of the time-dependent protoporphyrin IX concentration in normal human epidermis after delivery of ALA by passive topical application or iontophoresis. Photochem Photobiol 2002;75: 424–32.

36. Downie JB. Exploring the role for a new photodynamic cosmetic treatment. Pract Dermatol 2011; 8(9):50–1.

37. Gold MH, Biron JA. Safety and cosmetic effects of photodynamic therapy using hexyl aminolevulinate and intense pulsed light: a pilot study conducted in subjects with mild-to-moderate facial photodamage. J Clin Aesthet Dermatol 2013;6(10):27–31.

38. Chapas AM, Brightman I A, Weiss ET. Geronemus RGFacial rejuvenation using novel topical aminolevulinic acid ester. Presented at: American Academy of Dermatology Annual Meeting. New Orleans, February 4–8, 2011.

39. Moan J, Iani V, Ma L. Choice of the proper wavelength for photochemotherapy.

40. Smith S, Piacquadio D, Morhenn V, et al. Short incubation PDT versus 5-FU in treating actinic keratoses. J Drugs Dermatol 2003;2:629–35.

41. Arndt KA, Dover JS, Olbricht SM, editors. Lasers in cutaneous and aesthetic surgery. Philadelphia: Lippincott-Raven; 1997. p. 25–51.

42. Kalka K, Merk H, Mukhtar H. Photodynamic therapy in dermatology. J Am Acad Dermatol 2000; 42:389–413.

43. Clark C, Bryden A, Dawe R, et al. Topical 5- aminolaevulinic acid photodynamic therapy for cutaneous lesions: outcome and comparison of light sources. Photodermatol Photoimmunol Photomed 2003;19:134–41.

44. Friedmann DP, Goldman MP, Fabi SG, et al. The effect of multiple sequential light sources to activate aminolevulinic Acid in the treatment of actinic keratoses: a retrospective study. J Clin Aesthet Dermatol 2014;7:20–5.

45. Silva JN, Filipe P, Morliere P, et al. Photodynamic therapies: principles and present medical applications. Biomed Mater Eng 2006;16(4 Suppl): S147–54.

46. Lane KL, Hovenic W, Ball K, et al. Daylight photodynamic therapy: the Southern California experience. Lasers Surg Med 2015;47(2):168–72.

47. Kim M, Jung HY, Park HJ. Topical PDT in the treatment of benign skin diseases: principles and new applications. Int J Mol Sci 2015;16(10):23259–78.

48. Itoh Y1, Ninomiya Y, Tajima S, et al. Photodynamic therapy of acne vulgaris with topical delta-aminolaevulinic acid and incoherent light in Japanese patients. Br J Dermatol 2001;144(3):575–9.

49. Wiegell SR, Haedersdal M, Philipsen PA, et al. Continuous activation of PpIX by daylight is as effective as and less painful than conventional photodynamic therapy for actinic keratoses – a randomized, controlled, single-blinded study. Br J Dermatol 2008;158:740–6.

50. Wiegell SR, Hædersdal M, Eriksen P, et al. Photodynamic therapy of actinic keratoses with 8% and 16% methyl aminolevulinate and home-based daylight exposure: a double-blinded randomized clinical trial. Br J Dermatol 2009;160:1308–14.

51. Wiegell SR, Fabricius S, Stender IM, et al. A randomized, multicentre study of directed daylight exposure times of 1½ vs. 2½ h in daylight- mediated photodynamic therapy with methyl aminolevulinate in patients with multiple thin actinic keratoses of the face and scalp. Br J Dermatol 2011;164: 1083–90.

52. Wiegell SR, Wulf HC, Szeimies R-M, et al. Daylight photodynamic therapy for actinic keratosis: an international consensus. International Society for Photodynamic Therapy in Dermatology. J Eur Acad Dermatol Venereol 2012. https://doi.org/10. 1111/j.1468-3083.2011.04386.

53. Wulf HC, Pavel S, Stender I, et al. Topical photodynamic therapy for prevention of new skin lesions in renal transplant recipients. Acta Derm Venereol 2006;86:25–8.

54. Juzeniene A, Juzenas P, Kaalhus O, et al. Temperature effect on accumulation of protoporphyrin IX after topical application of 5-aminolevulinic acid and its methylester and hexylester derivatives in normal mouse skin. Photochem Photobiol 2002; 76:452–6.

55. Juzeniene A, Juzenas P, Bronshtein I, et al. The influence of temperature on photodynamic cell killing in vitro with 5-aminolevulinc acid. J Photochem Photobiol B 2006;84:161–6.

56. Hamblin MR, Hasan T. Photodynamic therapy: a new antimicrobial approach to infectious disease? Photochem Photobiol Sci 2004;3(5):436–50.

57. Dai T, Huang YY, Hamblin MR. Photodynamic therapy for localized infections–state of the art. Photodiagnosis Photodyn Ther 2009;6(3-4):170–88.

58. Kharkwal GB, Sharma SK, Huang YY, et al. Photodynamic therapy for infections: clinical applications. Lasers Surg Med 2011;43(7):755–67.

59. Konopka K, Goslinski T. Photodynamic therapy in dentistry. J Dent Res 2007;86:694.

60. Uhlenhake EE. Optimal treatment of actinic keratoses. Clin Interv Aging 2013;8:29–35.

61. Stern RS. Dermatologists and office-based care of dermatologic disease in the 21st century. J Investig Dermatol Symp Proc 2004;9(2):126–30.

62. Marks R, Rennie G, Selwood TS. Malignant transformation of solar keratoses to squamous cell carcinoma. Lancet 1988;1(8589):795–7.

63. Warino L, Tusa M, Camacho F, et al. Frequency and cost of actinic keratosis treatment. Dermatol Surg 2006;32(8):1045–9.

64. Haddican M, Goldenberg G. Update on the treatment of actinic keratoses. Wayne (PA): Bryn Mawr. Communications III LLC; 2012.

65. Lubritz RR, Smolewski SA. Cryosurgery cure rate of actinic keratoses. J Am Acad Dermatol 1982;7(5): 631–2.

66. Thai KE, Fergin P, Freeman M, et al. A prospective study of the use of cryosurgery for the treatment of actinic keratoses. Int J Dermatol 2004;43(9): 687–92.

67. McIntyre WJ, Downs MR, Bedwell SA. Treatment options for actinic keratoses. Am Fam Physician 2007;76(5):667–76.

68. Berman B, Cohen DE, Amini S. What is the role of field-directed therapy in the treatment of actinic keratosis? Part 1: overview and investigational topical agents. Cutis 2012;89(5):241–50.

69. Jeffes EW 3rd, Tang EH. Actinic keratosis. Current treatment options. Am J Clin Dermatol 2000;1(3): 167–79.

70. Alexiades-Armenakas MR, Geronemus RG. Laser-mediated photodynamic therapy for actinic keratoses. Arch Dermatol 2003;139(10):1313–20.

71. Salasche SJ. Epidemiology of actinic keratoses and squamous cell carcinoma. J Am Acad Dermatol 2000;42(1 Pt 2):4–7.

72. Stritt A, Merk HF, Braathen LR, et al. Photodynamic therapy in the treatment of actinic keratosis. Photochem Photobiol 2008;84(2):388–98.

73. Morton CA. Can photodynamic therapy reverse the signs of photoageing and field cancerization? Br J Dermatol 2012;167(1):2.

74. Tarstedt M, Rosdahl I, Berne B, et al. A randomized multicenter study to compare two treatment regimens of topical methyl aminolevulinate (Metvix)–PDT in actinic keratosis of the face and scalp. Acta Derm Venereol 2005;85(5):424–8.

75. Fuchs J, Thiele J. The role of oxygen in cutaneous photodynamic therapy. Free Radic Biol Med 1998; 24(5):835–47.

76. Kurwa HA, Yong-Gee SA, Seed PT, et al. A randomized paired comparison of photodynamic therapy and topical 5-fluorouracil in the treatment of actinic keratoses. J Am Acad Dermatol 1999; 41(3 Pt 1):414–8.

77. Patel G, Armstrong AW, Eisen DB. Efficacy of photodynamic therapy vs other interventions in randomized clinical trials for the treatment of actinic keratoses: a systematic review and meta-analysis. JAMA Dermatol 2014;150(12):1281–8.

78. Braathen LR, Szeimies RM, Basset-Seguin N, et al. Guidelines on the use of photodynamic therapy for nonmelanoma skin cancer: an international consensus. International Society for Photodynamic

Therapy in Dermatology, 2005. J Am Acad Dermatol 2007;56(1):125–43.

79. Kaufmann R, Spelman L, Weightman W, et al. Multicentre intraindividual randomized trial of topical methyl aminolaevulinate-photodynamic therapy vs. cryotherapy for multiple actinic keratoses on the extremities. Br J Dermatol 2008;158(5):994–9.

80. McLoone N, Donnelly RF, Walsh M, et al. Aminolaevulinic acid diffusion characteristics in 'in vitro' normal human skin and actinic keratosis: implications for topical photodynamic therapy. Photodermatol Photoimmunol Photomed 2008;24(4):183–90.

81. Tarstedt M, Gillstedt M, Wennberg Larkö AM, et al. Aminolevulinic acid and methyl aminolevulinate equally effective in topical photodynamic therapy for non-melanoma skin cancers. J Eur Acad Dermatol Venereol 2016;30(3):420–3.

82. Dirschka T, Radny P, Dominicus R, et al. Photodynamic therapy with BF-200 ALA for the treatment of actinic keratosis: results of a multicentre, randomized, observer-blind phase III study in comparison with a registered methyl-5-aminolaevulinate cream and placebo. Br J Dermatol 2012;166(1): 137–46.

83. Dirschka T, Radny P, Dominicus R, et al. Long-term (6 and 12 months) follow-up of two prospective, randomized, controlled phase III trials of photodynamic therapy with BF-200 ALA and methyl aminolaevulinate for the treatment of actinic keratosis. Br J Dermatol 2013;168(4):825–36.

84. Gholam P, Weberschock T, Denk K, et al. Treatment with 5-aminolaevulinic acid methylester is less painful than treatment with 5-aminolaevulinic acid nanoemulsion in topical photodynamic therapy for actinic keratosis. Dermatology 2011;222(4): 358–62.

85. Farrell LN, Strauss JS, Stranieri AM. The treatment of severe cystic acne with 13-cis-retinoic acid: evaluation of sebum production and the clinical response in a multiple-dose trial. J Am Acad Dermatol 1980;3(6):602–11.

86. Thielitz A1, Gollnick H. Topical retinoids in acne vulgaris: update on efficacy and safety. Am J Clin Dermatol 2008;9(6):369–81.

87. Chandrashekar BS, Ashwini KR, Vasanth V, et al. Retinoic acid and glycolic acid combination in the treatment of acne scars. Indian Dermatol Online J 2015;6(2):84–8.

88. Sharad J. Glycolic acid peel therapy - a current review. Clin Cosmet Investig Dermatol 2013;6:281–8.

89. Atzori L, Brundu MA, Orru A, et al. Glycolic acid peeling in the treatment of acne. J Eur Acad Dermatol Venereol 1999;12(2):119–22.

90. Moy LS. Superficial chemical peels with alpha-hydroxy acids. In: Robinson JK, Arndt KA, Le Boit PE, et al, editors. Atlas of cutaneous surgery. Philadelphia: WB Saunders; 1996. p. 345–50.

91. Moy LS, Murad H, Moy RL. Glycolic acid peels for the treatment of wrinkles and photoaging. J Dermatol Surg Oncol 1993;19(3):243–6.

92. Bernstein EF, Lee J, Brown DB, et al. Glycolic acid treatment increases type I collagen mRNA and hyaluronic acid content of human skin. Dermatol Surg 2001;27(5):429–33.

93. Boen M, Brownell J, Patel P, et al. The role of photodynamic therapy in acne: an evidence-based review. Am J Clin Dermatol 2017;18(3): 311–21.

94. Riddle CC, Terrell SN, Menser MB, et al. A review of photodynamic therapy (PDT) for the treatment of acne vulgaris. J Drugs Dermatol 2009;8(11): 1010–9.

95. Fabbrocini G, Cacciapuoti S, De Vita V, et al. The effect of aminolevulinic acid photodynamic therapy on microcomedones and macrocomedones. Dermatology 2009;219(4):322–8.

96. Yin R, Hao F, Deng J, et al. Investigation of optimal aminolaevulinic acid concentration applied in topical aminolaevulinic acid-photodynamic therapy for treatment of moderate to severe acne: a pilot study in Chinese subjects. Br J Dermatol 2010; 163(5):1064–71.

97. Ma L, Xiang LH, Yu B, et al. Low-dose topical 5-aminolevulinic acid photodynamic therapy in the treatment of different severity of acne vulgaris. Photodiagnosis Photodyn Ther 2013;10(4): 583–90.

98. Wiegell SR, Wulf HC. Photodynamic therapy of acne vulgaris using 5-aminolevulinic acid versus methyl aminolevulinate. J Am Acad Dermatol 2006;54(4):647–51.

99. Song BH, Lee DH, Kim BC, et al. Photodynamic therapy using chlorophyll-a in the treatment of acne vulgaris: a randomized, single-blind, split-face study. J Am Acad Dermatol 2014;71(4): 76471.

100. Na JI, Kim SY, Kim JH, et al. Indole-3-acetic acid: a potential new photosensitizer for photodynamic therapy of acne vulgaris. Lasers Surg Med 2011; 43(3):200–5.

101. Handler MZ, Bloom BS, Goldberg DJ. Energy-based devices in treatment of acne vulgaris. Dermatol Surg 2016;42(5):573–85.

102. Tzung TY, Wu KH, Huang ML. Blue light phototherapy in the treatment of acne. Photodermatol Photoimmunol Photomed 2004;20(5):266–9.

# Moving?

## Make sure your subscription moves with you!

To notify us of your new address, find your **Clinics Account Number** (located on your mailing label above your name), and contact customer service at:

**Email: journalscustomerservice-usa@elsevier.com**

**800-654-2452** (subscribers in the U.S. & Canada)
**314-447-8871** (subscribers outside of the U.S. & Canada)

**Fax number: 314-447-8029**

**Elsevier Health Sciences Division**
**Subscription Customer Service**
**3251 Riverport Lane**
**Maryland Heights, MO 63043**

Printed and bound by CPI Group (UK) Ltd, Croydon, CR0 4YY

08/05/2025

01864746-0017